Dr Torkil Færø is a general practitioner and emergency physician, documentary filmmaker, author and photographer. In 1996 he was one of the first Norwegian medics to work for Doctors Without Borders when he worked in war-torn Angola. Over a 25-year career as a freelance doctor, he has worked all over Norway, had tens of thousands of consultations and gained a unique picture of the diseases that plague us. He has learned that the cause is most often found in the stresses our lifestyles place on our bodies.

Færø is also an award-winning photographer, author of *Kamerakuren* (*The Camera Cure*), and has made documentaries about his pilgrimages to Nidaros and Santiago de Compostela. An inveterate traveller, he has made his way by bicycle, motorbike, kayak, sailboat and car through over 80 countries, and speaks eight languages. He lives in Oslo with his wife and two children.

Praise for *The Pulse Cure*

'*The Pulse Cure* is a groundbreaking exploration of how HRV data can revolutionise our approach to health. As an immunologist, I appreciate the depth of insight provided in this book, which bridges the gap between cutting-edge science and practical well-being. A must-read for anyone seeking to improve their immune resilience, reduce inflammation and embrace a healthier future.'

Dr Jenna Macciochi, author of *Immunity: The Science of Staying Well*

'The Pulse Cure and HRV is a health revolution!'

Dr Annette Dragland, doctor and presenter of *Doctors on Life*

'Do you want to get more out of everyday life? Then you should read *The Pulse Cure*. Dr Torkil Færø covers everything you need to know and understand about how you can easily reduce your stress level with the help of a heart rate monitor. He gives you simple and effective tools that can help you find peace, balance and, above all, a healthier life. A revolutionary book that I hope many will read.'

Dr Carina Saunders, paediatrician, researcher and author

'You can actually learn what affects the nervous system positively and what affects the nervous system negatively. You may not want to be online with your own body for the rest of your life, but for a period of months you will learn what adds and what depletes energy in your life. Not least it will teach you to take measures in time so that you get enough rest and enough positive input in your everyday life so you can avoid burnout.'

Egil Arne Skaun Knutsen, psychologist

'Fantastic read! Færø is at the forefront of an exciting change in how we relate to our health.'

Dr Herman Egenberg, doctor and presenter of the podcast *Motivational Interview*

'*The Pulse Cure* is ground-breaking and will provide revolutionary knowledge for all practitioners who provide healthcare.'

Annette Løno, neuroflexologist

'As a doctor with a special interest in stress and mindfulness, it is wonderful to read *The Pulse Cure*. It is inspiring, professionally sound and opens up a whole new landscape for how both private individuals and healthcare professionals can learn to measure HRV and the autonomic nervous system. Recommended for healthcare professionals and anyone else who wants to learn a new tool to biohack their own health.'

Ragnhild Skari Luell, doctor and mindfulness instructor

'Lots of inspiration with engagingly communicated knowledge and excellent, concrete help for anyone who wants to make informed choices for their own mental and physical health.

The Pulse Cure is suitable for anyone who is curious about how they can get more mental and physical surplus and energy in everyday life, and how they can make good choices that promote their own health . . . Even the experienced can learn new tools that can contribute to better health.'

Gry Husebø, psychologist

'Torkil Færø shows us how we can facilitate a good balance between stress and rest in our own body – and in our own life. He explains complex phenomena in an easily understandable and entertaining way, and through examples and practical exercises, invites us to get to know our own wonderful nervous system better. This is a book that I think many people will benefit from and enjoy.'

Inger Tone Kleven, psychologist

'An easy-to-understand book that takes individual needs seriously. The strength of *The Pulse Cure* lies in the individual perspective. It is an easily accessible tool both for those who want to stay healthy and for those who are looking for ways to get healthier.'

Dr Erik Hexeberg, specialist in internal medicine and author

'A game changer! *The Pulse Cure* is a real page-turner and a joy to read: entertaining, informative and well written . . . I look forward to showing my patients how they can benefit from using a smartwatch to support them in making good choices for their health and well-being.'

Kristin Bothner Kanstad, MD, specialist in general medicine and psychiatry, yoga and mindfulness teacher

'*The Pulse Cure* shows you how to interpret what the heart rate monitor shows, and how the pulse variation affects your health. When you understand these connections, it's easier to make the good lifestyle changes you know you need!'

Dr Gunhild Melleby, psychiatrist

'What *The Pulse Cure* has taught me about balancing the autonomic nervous system has given me back my night's sleep after several decades of sleep deprivation. In addition, the knowledge is a fantastic addition to my work with managers who struggle with burnout! Torkil Færø will probably contribute to a significant health-promoting shift in society's view of the value of restitution.'

Heddy Anne Torp Lund, Coach and Gestalt psychotherapist

'*The Pulse Cure* is . . . a welcome and appreciated contribution among the flood of health books. Færø has done a formidable job of summarising this topic in ways that patients and the general public will greatly benefit from.

Færø has done important pioneering work in systematically exploring and presenting his own and his test group's experiences.

I hope that not only "most people" but all Norwegian doctors read *The Pulse Cure* and familiarise themselves with how to influence their stress and inflammation levels through lifestyle interventions.'

Iver Mysterud, *Helsemagasinet* (*The Health Magazine*)

THE PULSE CURE

BALANCE STRESS, OPTIMISE
HEALTH AND LIVE LONGER

DR TORKIL FÆRØ

QUERCUS

First published in Norway in 2023
under the title *Pulskuren* by Cappelen Damm As, Oslo.
This translation first published in Great Britain by

QUERCUS

Quercus Editions Ltd
Carmelite House
50 Victoria Embankment
London EC4Y 0DZ

An Hachette UK company

English language edition published in agreement with
NORTHERN STORIES. (All rights reserved)
English translation by Robert Moses

The author has received support from the Non-fiction Fund to write this book.

A CIP catalogue record for this book is available
from the British Library

TPB ISBN 9781529437331
Ebook ISBN 9781529437348

10 9 8 7 6 5 4 3

Typeset by Jouve (UK), Milton Keynes

Printed and bound in Great Britain by Clays Ltd, Elcograf S.p.A.

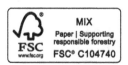

Papers used by Quercus are from well-managed forests and other responsible sources.

In loving memory of my father Tore Færø (1940–2013), whose too-early death inspired me to change my lifestyle.

Contents

Contents

The doctor of the future will be oneself.

Albert Schweitzer, German doctor, theologian,
organist, musicologist, and philosopher

Join this expedition!

Imagine there was an instrument that could measure your stress levels and show you how much stress your body can take. It could give you an indication when you should slow down and relax to regain the balance between stress and relaxation in your life, and could help you gain a surplus of energy for you to call on every day. It could measure how much willpower you have at your disposal. It could tell you when you have recharged your batteries during the night while you slept. It could educate you as to when is the best time to eat before ending your day and make you aware of to what extent alcohol impacts your ability to function the day after drinking. It could determine exactly how much *you* should work out and how long you need to recover from it afterwards. It could give you the answer as to when is the right time to go back to work after being away on sick leave. It could give you the tools you need to turn back your biological clock. And, finally, it could reveal to you if you have pathogenic inflammation in your body almost immediately and whether there is a risk of it developing into a serious illness. This tool would be affordable and portable, and it could help you to get better control over your health and to live a healthier and longer life.

This instrument and its applications are not in fact part of some distant dream taking place in the future or something that is too good to be true. This monitoring tool does exist, and, in this book, you will learn how to use it. We need something like this because in our day and age the balance of our stress is out of whack. Many people get ill from eating badly, becoming overly stressed out, and sleeping too little, and they lack the means to achieve a state of inner calm and peace of mind. Other people fall ill for the opposite reasons. They give themselves too few challenges and would prefer just to relax even after they are fully rested, thus passively allowing their bodies and minds to deteriorate.

The right stress balance increases our willpower in any given moment as well as our capacity to function. It also improves the overall quality of our lives. It gives us a better state of health, resistance to disease, and a longer life.

I would like to invite you to embark on an exciting expedition. Together, we will take a deep dive into humanity's ancient, self-regulating nervous system and learn how it can be tamed through the aid of modern technology. It is a journey that I have undertaken myself and I would love to be your guide along the way.

Anita (58)
The Pulse Cure has taught me a lot and given me the tools I need to be able to regulate and balance stress in my life. I now make more conscious choices when it comes to sleeping, eating, scheduling my meals, drinking alcohol, exercising, and being active as well as resting and recovering. Working with this book has improved my health and quality of life.

PLANNING YOUR EXPEDITION

Whereas a casual trip can be spontaneous, meandering and require little effort, for an expedition you need to plan. First, we first need to know what goal we are moving towards. Then we need to prepare, so that we have the knowledge and tools we will need and are ready for any challenges we may encounter along the way.

Our goal

The primary aim of this expedition is to discover how to find your optimal stress balance by managing your autonomic (self-regulating) nervous system. To achieve this, you will learn how to use a heart rate monitor.

The autonomic nervous system that each of us carries within us regulates the body's basic functions and has survived for millions of years. Unlike our conscious, thought-controlled brains, our unconscious nervous system has no notion that we live in the 2020s. Nor does it differentiate between a human being and a reptile. Our bodies and brains have the same need for stress regulation, rest, and sleep, as any other vertebrate that we share this planet with.

If it weren't for all the health problems we now suffer from, we could leave our nervous systems to operate in secret, but our modern lifestyle is wearing them down. We are overly busy, rest too little and sleep too little, are too sedentary, eat badly, and make ourselves ill with stress. Our bodies and minds are being stretched to breaking point; we were never designed for today's tempo and rhythm of life. Living with artificial light means that we are active for longer hours and sleep less than previous generations did. We have invented transport methods and technological conveniences that result in us moving around less. And the rise of information technology has led to our being constantly connected, so that our brains rarely get to switch off.

There is now a fundamental conflict between society's demands and how the human body and brain are constructed. Yet, although many of the lifestyle diseases of our time are influenced by societal pressures, we are all, ultimately, responsible for our own lives. We may not be to blame for the problem, but we can take ownership of it. Rather than waiting for society to change, we must change ourselves. It's easier and faster.

And a heart rate monitor can increase the chances of our success.

The aim of measuring your pulse is to better understand your autonomic nervous system, and so have more flexibility in how you manage your energy. You will then find calm in your body more easily when it's needed or mobilise your forces for life's tougher moments when they arise. Recording these measurements is not an end in itself; it is a means by which you can revolutionise your life with greater inner resources and strength to enjoy existence and fulfil your dreams.

Your guide

If I was going on an expedition, I would want to know something about my guide, so let me tell you a little about myself. As I write this, I am a 53-year-old doctor, photographer, documentary filmmaker, and author. I live in Oslo, Norway, with my wife and two teenaged children.

My motivation for becoming a doctor was perhaps a little different from that of many of my colleagues. I wanted to have a front-row seat on life – to observe the stages of life we all go through close up and to participate in the lives of as many people as I could. Being a doctor has allowed me to do this. As a general practitioner and an A&E emergency physician I deal with people from before they are born and until after they have died. I have taken splinters out of people's fingers and toes and have looked into thousands of ears. And I have also been through countless dramatic situations where people's lives are on the line and in which the decisions I make can have major consequences. My experiences with patients over the length of an entire generation have formed an important foundation for this book.

I also wanted to pack as many experiences into this one life as I could. Being a doctor has given me the freedom to work when and where I desired. From 1999 until the present time I have worked in 30 municipalities throughout Norway, ranging from the south to the north, along fjords and in the mountains, and in cities and rural areas. And while working for Doctors Without Borders in war-torn Angola in 1996, I gained insight into the reality of the healthcare sector worldwide.

By working intensively for weeks at a time, I freed up time to discover and experience other countries and people, and at the same time develop the hobbies I like doing, such as photography and sailing around the world. My love of photography, desire to travel, and restlessness were too great for me to be able to combine them with a fixed position in the healthcare system.

I have published a book about photography, *Kamerakuren* (*The Camera Cure*), and have also made two documentary films for the Norwegian Broadcasting Corporation (NRK) about pilgrimages, one to Nidaros Cathedral in Trondheim, Norway, and one to Santiago de Compostela, Spain. To my great delight, these TV films have inspired many people to embark on healthy and life-enhancing walks. In fact, they may have contributed to as many positive health outcomes for people as the efforts I have made at my medical practice.

As a doctor, I feel a growing discomfort in my role as someone who is supposed to diagnose, prescribe medication, and refer patients for a myriad of tests, examinations, and specialised care. The way we practise medicine is backwards: we wait until people become ill before we 'heroically' intervene. It is as if we continue to retrieve badly injured people from the bottom of a valley with a helicopter and use all the hospital's technology and human resources to save them instead of installing safety barriers that could have prevented them from falling in the first place, thereby averting the whole disaster. Preventative medicine is a kind of safety barrier and monitoring our heart rate variability is a key element for practising it.

To some extent, people's bad health choices have given me a career; they have paid for things like my apartment and sailing around the world, but it would have been nice to practise progressive medicine that centred around maintaining people's health. I hope that this book can help to keep you *away* from the doctor.

But perhaps my most important credential for writing this book is this: I myself have made all the mistakes that I write about here. It is a journey I have made personally. Far from being a strict, preachy, know-it-all expert speaking from atop his high horse, I have the same compassion for you as I do for the person I was for many years.

My hope is to be able to convey my accumulated knowledge in an inspiring way and contribute to you being able to have a healthier, better-balanced life as well as enjoying increased vitality.

Right, now you know a little about my experience, let's get started.

Getting ready

The secret to any successful expedition lies in good preparation. So, we'll start in your armchair, or any other place from which you are comfortable to study the theory that lies behind our planned journey. First, you will be given a good grounding in physiology, the brain, the autonomic nervous system, and the immune system, and how the hitherto unknown body budget can be balanced.

You will also learn about the instruments we plan to use to track our journey. Instead of GPS, a map, and a compass, you will need just one instrument: *a heart rate monitor*. What this is, and how it is used, you will soon find out. But before you start taking any readings, I would advise you to spend a little time on the theory which I will present here. You will then be equipped to make better decisions later in your expedition.

The long path to getting control over the autonomic nervous system is divided into several manageable stages. How long each one takes will depend on the challenges you experience along the way, and how much effort you put in.

This whole book takes an estimated five hours to read, and during these 20,000 heartbeats and 4,000 breaths you will hopefully have made an investment in millions more of them!

The process

Equipped with your preferred heart rate monitor, you will investigate how different factors affect your autonomic nervous system. The sooner you see the results, the more easily you can make good choices.

I cannot promise it will be easy, although the techniques you learn here will help. If it were really easy to get healthy, everyone would be fit, slim, energetic, and strong. But it's even harder if we do *not* take care of ourselves. Over time this can lead to years of crippling ailments and illnesses.

I will try to make your journey to health as easy and pleasurable as possible. There can in fact be a lot of joy in discovering and exploring oneself and consequently in working towards becoming a stronger, more balanced, and strong-willed person. In short, this means taking control of one's own health.

I promise to use as few theoretical words and concepts as possible. My aim is to equip you with sufficient information to enable you to optimise your nervous system in the simplest way possible.

> **Synnøve (38)**
> I have found out that living a simple and natural lifestyle, which includes getting enough rest and avoiding being bound to a packed schedule and saying 'yes' to everything that pops up, provides a rock-solid foundation for keeping me staying lively and in good health. We have to adjust our day according to the amount of energy we have. I never learnt on my own how to find this out but now, with the help of being able to measure my heart rate variability, I am aware of it!

A caveat before we begin

When I was studying medicine, my lecturers always emphasised two things:

1. Medicine is not an exact science: the body's 'universe' is so diverse and complex that it is not possible to get a full overview of it and it is difficult to find exact answers to questions about it.
2. Medical facts have a half-life of five years: what we once believed to be true now proves to be false, and what will turn out to be correct at some point has not been discovered yet.

I believe that we should approach science and our application of it with humility since even medical facts are in constant development. This is particularly true in the preventative health field that I am now writing about. The amount and breadth of knowledge in this area has taken off only in the last decade, and our understanding will only deepen in the years to come. It is therefore important to read this book as a guide and not as a bible. The advice in this book should not replace the guidance you would get from your own doctor who, when it comes down to it, has the best knowledge about your medical condition. Nor would I recommend that anyone stop taking their regular medications without first consulting with a doctor.

The stages

I have divided the steps that are needed for balancing your stress and having a longer and healthier life into stages:

1. You learn about **sleep** and how the quality of it can be improved.
2. You learn about **stress** and how you can find a sustainable, productive level of it.
3. You find a level of **movement** and **exercise** that suits you that promotes good health.
4. You explore different ways of **resting** and establishing **calm** within.
5. You learn how **food** impacts your physiology.
6. You discover why **alcohol** can be considered 'liquid stress'.
7. You experience how **illnesses and diseases** can be detected in your heart rate variability.
8. You learn about the significance of being **overweight.**
9. You find out about how **smoking** and the use of **tobacco** products affects the nervous system.

I am happy that you are seizing this opportunity to come along on this expedition. It will decrease the chances of meeting you at my doctor's practice. I am sure that you are a nice, interesting person and that it would be a pleasure to get to know you, but I would prefer that you stay healthy. In my experience, a very large proportion of the illnesses I treat are rooted in an imbalance in the autonomic nervous system. Put another way, they can be prevented.

The path to better health is measurable and accessible to everyone. Even though reaching your goal may be way up ahead in front of you, this journey starts with the first step. Appreciating the hardships we encounter along the way increases our chances of reaching that goal.

Very rarely do I treat people who are worn out because they have exerted themselves for the sake of improving themselves. On the contrary, I treat many patients for the exact opposite: they are tired because they have *not* made any efforts to improve their health. So, instead of having pity for you, this book is full of tough love. Together, we must keep our eyes fixed on the process of recovery. Let's embark on this expedition equipped with an enthusiasm for life itself and appreciate the fact that we have options that our great-grandparents could only dream of, as well as a standard of living that just a few generations ago would have been reserved for royalty. Take good care of your unique opportunity for a long, healthy, and exciting life!

THE TERMS I USE IN THIS BOOK

As you read you might wonder: 'What is meant by physiology?' Physiology is just one of several central terms you might as well get to know now rather than later. They will appear throughout the book and will eventually be more fully explained. If you forget what a word or expression means, then just return to this brief introduction.

1. The autonomic nerve system
2. Physiology
3. Heart rate variability
4. Heart rate monitor
5. Body budget

The autonomic nervous system

The autonomic (self-regulating) nervous system, which is the ancient, inner living fossil that we share with all vertebrates, is the body's hidden drivetrain. It is well-hidden inside of us and it is often overlooked by the healthcare system as well as by most people. That's a shame because, from my experience of meeting with thousands of patients, imbalances in the body's basic physiological processes often lead to a reduced quality of life, unnecessary illness, and an early death.

The autonomic nervous system, among other things, regulates our stress levels, alertness, circadian rhythm, digestion, heart rate, breathing rate, inflammation levels, immune system, and energy balance, including blood sugar level and fat metabolism. The system consists of the activating *sympathetic* nervous system, which mobilises the body and the brain, and the calming *parasympathetic* system, which sees to the body's recovery and restitution. This division (with an on-off function splitting them) can be found in most organisms and this inheritance is something we should consider more if we want to maintain our health. For our bodies to function well, we need to be able to mobilise energies within ourselves and to make sure that we get enough rest. A heart rate monitor can help us to preserve this balance.

Physiology

One's physiology is a sort of overall picture of the body's basic functioning, from the smallest cellular processes to the entire biochemical balance of the body. Almost everything here runs on autopilot, but the activities we do, as well as our thoughts, have an enormous effect on the various processes taking place within us. Whereas the subject of anatomy names the different parts that make up the body, physiology sheds light on how the different parts function throughout one's life. For example, a dead person's anatomy will remain intact even though his or her physiological processes have stopped.

The autonomic nervous system is the foundation stone that regulates much of the activity in our complex physiology. A serious imbalance in our physiology will easily result in psychological or physical symptoms. Often, we ask ourselves if something happening to us has psychological or physical roots. However, I think we would benefit from asking ourselves whether the cause might be physiological. As soon as we have made sure that our physiology is in balance then we can return to asking ourselves the original question if the symptoms persist as before.

Heart rate variability

Our pulse reveals whether our autonomic nervous system is in balance, and it shows us the degree of stress on the body. When you are in a state of rest, i.e. when the nervous system is in the de-stressed parasympathetic state, the distance between heartbeats will vary during inhalation or exhalation. Your pulse will quicken when you inhale, to exploit the fact that your lungs are filled with oxygen, and then slow down when you exhale, to save energy, much like a wave in the ocean that crests quickly followed by a longer trough. When that is the case, your pulse variation, also known as *heart rate variability* (HRV), is high.

When you are in a state of stress, i.e. when the nervous system is in the sympathetic, mobilised mode, then your lungs will contain less oxygen and your body cannot afford to lower its heart rate during exhalation. As a result, there will be less variation in the distance between heartbeats. The heart will then beat more like a clock. In other words, your heart rate variability will be low, and it will result in you being stressed. As you will see in this book, the cause of what we perceive as stress can be more than just being busy or mentally restless. Stress whose cause appears hidden to us also occurs due to a lack of sleep, eating meals late in the evening, exercising, alcohol, and several other factors.

We need a good balance between time spent being in the stress and resting modes. An imbalance between these two will result in physical and psychological issues. A balanced nervous system gives us a surplus of energy and willpower. Your heart rate variability is a biomarker, a measurement of the degree of physical as well as psychological illness present in the body, as well as the probability of being afflicted by one.

Heart rate monitor

In the past, we needed knowledgeable personnel to handle large, complex devices in order to show us tiny changes in our pulse down to the millisecond. In recent years, however, advanced, easily accessible technology has been developed that can register our heart rate variability on smartphones, rings, bracelets, and chest monitors. Even a mobile phone camera in combination with the light on the phone can be used. These technological tools are available in a wide range of prices and in several varieties, from simple measurement devices to sophisticated systems that can guide you individually.

A heart rate monitor is a kind of physiological speedometer that records whether your tempo is sustainable over a period of time. In addition to reading this book, user-friendly apps on smartphones can also provide you with good guidance. In other words, it is possible for you to measure your body's autonomic nervous system on your own.

And what we can measure, we can more easily master!

> **Lena (59)**
> Initially, I was very sceptical of heart rate monitors, but after some time I have pretty much become an ambassador on their behalf. A heart rate monitor gives me a certain overview of how my body is doing and what considerations I should take when it is not doing so well. You know, it doesn't really help much to tell yourself to 'just pull yourself together and get on with it' and then start self-flagellating when in fact the only thing the body really needs is some peace and rest.

Body budget

Each of us has a certain amount of physiological energy that is available to us to be used for physical and mental tasks. I call it a *body budget*. Our job is to try to balance this budget and hopefully have a little energy left over. When it comes to a big variation in our heart rate – that is, when we are in the parasympathetic, resting mode – our body battery is being recharged and the budget receives what can be considered capital. With a small variation in heart rate, when we are doing an activity that mobilises the sympathetic nervous system, we drain the battery. We use energy from the same account regardless of what the stress was that activated the sympathetic part of the nervous system – it could be a fight with your partner, a rather large meal, two glasses of wine, or a workout. Everything is connected to everything else, especially when it comes to the body.

Our heart rate variability can show us if we have drained or replenished our body budget. Heart rate monitor apps reveal how much is going into and out of our physiological account and how much spare energy we have to work with at any given time.

Just as we have bank statements and online banking for keeping track of the state of our financial affairs, so we can use heart rate monitors to keep an eye on our physiological energy balance sheet, whether it relates to our outgoings or our income at a given moment, or looking at what's been accrued over a given period of time. Though it is certainly important to balance our finances, it is absolutely vital to balance our physiology!

> **Synnøve (38)**
> It is so simple and valuable! Looking at the data for the Body Battery ought to be just as natural for us to do as checking the battery on our mobile phones. Comparing how you feel with the Body Battery numbers displayed on a watch is a useful tool for being more aware of your health.

THE TEST GROUP'S TERMINOLOGY

While working on this book, I involved a working group consisting of 198 people. They used Garmin watches to measure their heart rate variability and consequently they acquired an overview of their body budget. The participants were recruited after I appeared as a guest on the Norwegian podcast *Leger om livet* (*Doctors on Life*) in March 2022. Their efforts have been invaluable. Spread throughout this book you can read their testimonials, which illustrate what they have learnt by working with heart rate monitors. You will come across two terms:

1. *Body Battery (BB)*, which is Garmin's measurement of the physiological resources you currently have available (either the body battery or body budget). The scale measuring it goes from 5 to 100 in which 5 is the lowest value and 100 means the battery is full.
2. *Stress*, which is Garmin's measurement for the amount of stress you are experiencing in a given moment. The reading is in blue while in the resting mode and orange in the stress mode. The scale here goes from 0 to 100 in which 0 is the lowest of stress and 100 is the highest.

I hope that the input from the test group will be both educational and inspirational as we move ahead!

BUT WHAT ABOUT YOU?

I have given you an idea as to who I am, and what we are here for. Now, I am going to have a guess as to who you are.

I am very curious about who you are! The only thing I do know about you is that you are interested in improving your health and that you have enough initiative to take some active steps to make it happen. You, after all, have either bought or borrowed this book. You want to acquire more knowledge about your physiological condition so you can improve it. And now that you have read this far, you have revealed that you have a drive and an ability to carry things out that I would like to help you maintain.

So, who are you?

I am going to take a shot in the dark and guess that you belong to one of the four following categories: Exhausted, Hanging on, Healthy, or Helper.

1. **Exhausted:** You have felt how your body and mind can fail you when you need it the most. You have spent time seeing doctors and health-care professionals and have tried several different treatment methods to improve your health. The symptoms, such as fatigue, mood swings, muscular and skeletal problems, stomach pain, restlessness, anxiety, depression, sleep difficulties, headaches, and dizziness can vary. These symptoms are often a sign that the body is in a general state of inflammation, and you may be taking medication for a number of these conditions. This is the category of people I know the best. Half of my working day at my practice is filled with addressing these issues. Health problems reduce your capacity to function well and destroy your joie de vivre: you often have problems mobilising your will-power and making changes. Unfortunately, I know all too well how difficult it is to find methods or treatments that can be of help. Measuring your heart rate variability could be life-changing for you. It might be that your autonomic nervous system is on the edge of being broken down. Getting it back on track may require a huge effort in terms of making lifestyle changes and you just may need to work together with a therapist or a doctor who is knowledgeable about heart rate variability in order to succeed in doing so.

2. **Hanging on:** You function well in life and at work but feel like your petrol tank is nearly empty. You get tired periodically and have some physical symptoms but contact the healthcare system only sporadically. Maybe you have suffered from one or two chronic illnesses and use a couple of medications regularly. You have realised that parts of your lifestyle are not benefitting you and you would like some help to improve your health and have a surplus of energy. You have an idea that adjustments in your levels of activity, relaxation, the food you eat, and your sleep will help you. I am also quite familiar with people in this category. In fact, for many years this was me. You will be able to get good results quickly and get into balance with some gradual, small changes and will be encouraged by actually seeing the results of your efforts. You will probably be able to figure all of this out on your own, or perhaps in collaboration with a friend. Possibly, you will need a visit or two to a doctor or a therapist. Your changes in lifestyle will greatly reduce your risk of disease, a decreased quality of life, and the shortening of your lifespan. Your new surplus of energy will not only benefit you but also the people around you.

3. **Healthy:** You function well both at home and at work and do not have any significant health problems. But maybe your family history indicates that you have an increased risk for contracting certain diseases and you want to take preventative measures. Or maybe you have some ambitions or a job or an all-consuming interest that require that your body and mind function optimally. You need all the energy you can muster at your disposal to be able to follow your dreams and achieve the goals you set for yourself. You also want to have a little something extra to draw upon in case life throws a curveball in the form of a divorce, illness, or other unexpected stressful situation. Maybe you are simply just curious about this new tool and want to find out if it could be useful for you? You would, undoubtedly, experience great benefits from having better control over your physiology and so introducing a more joyful, pleasurable flow into your life. After all, we do not have to be in a poor state of health in order to want to improve it!

Increased mental and physical capacities can help you have the willpower to reach your goals. Perhaps you could team up with a like-minded, motivated friend?

4. **Helper:** You are one of the many people who work to help others to make improvements. Perhaps you yourself have managed to get sufficient control over your own physiology after a long period when you did not have it? You have learnt this knowledge and now you want to work in the role of passing it on. Maybe you are a yoga instructor, meditation teacher, fitness instructor, doctor, psychologist, or life coach? Or you have one of the many other occupations that involve helping people to have a better life. Heart rate monitors could be an important tool for you in your work. Feel free, though, to use a heart rate monitor to take care of *your* health. We helpers who work with people facing difficulties are the occupational group who are most at risk for getting burnt out. We have to have our feet planted on solid ground to be able to help others get up.

I wrote this book for you regardless of which of the four categories you find yourself in – or even if none of these groups resonates with you! Taking control over one's physiology is important for each and every one of us, regardless of whether we are currently healthy or so unwell that we can hardly keep our heads above water. It does not matter whether you feel sick, just so-so, or healthy – you can always improve your health.

Vibeke (49)
My health has been on a downward trajectory since 2003 and I've been suffering from extreme fatigue since 2018. I have grown worse and worse and have struggled with trying to slow down my level of activity and exercising. Keeping track of my heart rate variability with the monitor gives me a framework for disciplining myself and now I have a much better grasp of how much I in fact need to rest in order to achieve a sustainable balance between activity and rest.

YOUR GOALS, VALUES AND DREAMS

You have now gained a little insight into this expedition that we are about to set off on. I would class this as a classic hero's journey, one where epic obstacles will be encountered before a great reward is earned. However, the obstacles are not in the way, they *are* the way. Through encountering and dealing with them we make ourselves more resilient and hardier.

So, now we're going to write down our goals, values, and dreams. A person who knows their short-term goals, personal values, and long-term dreams will be more able to stay the course. Maybe it seems strange to have to do such a formal exercise, but seeing the words on the page will both make your thoughts clearer to you and obligate you to follow through. Go ahead and put your signature at the bottom of the form to help drive it home that you really mean business. Then take it one step at a time. Every single little step in the right direction will inspire you to take new steps and will be essential for any future breakthrough. The Pareto principle is applicable here: 20% of the efforts you make will lead to 80% of the results. In other words, a little goes a long way and doing something, anything, can turn out to be just enough. Prioritise small changes in several areas rather than one big change restricted to only one.

My goals, values, and dreams

1. What is your goal? What do you specifically want to get out of working with this book?

   • _____

2. What are your values? Whereas your goal says something about *what* you want to achieve, a clarification of your values will tell you *why* you want to do it. I want to be a person who:

   • _____
   • _____
   • _____
   • _____

3. What dreams do you have for your life in the future? List five of them below. Reminding yourself about them may be of help should your motivation wane along the way. I will:

- _____
- _____
- _____
- _____
- _____

I promise to do my best so that this expedition is a success.

I promise to lead this expedition in a positive, satisfying, and safe manner so that you can experience a better balance in your life regarding stress and have better health for a longer period of time as well as having the greatest possible chance of reaching your goals.

_____
Date and your signature

_____
Torkil Færø

Yngvar (47)
I lived a wonderful life in which I was much in demand. Positive reports about my lectures literally spread from Alta, Norway, to San Francisco. I had designed a carefree life for myself both privately and at work in which I exclusively did things that I liked doing and was good at, together with people I valued highly. I spent a lot of time flying, going through a lot of airports, and eating a lot of late meals, followed by a lot of great parties afterwards. I didn't have any stress in my life, or so I thought. But one day my body gave out. I became

exhausted and dizzy. My heart pounded quickly and hard, there was a prickling sensation in my arms, and sometimes I could not feel my own skin. At its worst, all I could manage was to marshal my energy for 45 minutes in the morning to make breakfast and lunch for my kids to take with them to school before crashing back into bed. A psychologist, my GP, and a physiotherapist eventually agreed on a diagnosis: *an overdose of positive stress*. The physiotherapist tipped me off about the *Leger om livet* (*Doctors on Life*) podcast in which Torkil Færø was a guest. This led me to begin measuring my heart rate variability with a monitor.

I made dramatic changes. I cancelled all my travels for two months, began sleeping longer, meditated, cut down my alcohol consumption to very little, and was ruthless when it came to prioritising which work assignments and social activities I would say yes to.

I began living what would, by most estimates, be considered a clean, moderate lifestyle (think: drinking half a glass of wine alongside an excellent meal) and I was sleeping an average of nine hours a night. After a month of this, I managed to be 'nearly recovered' (all the experts were in agreement about this) astonishingly quickly. Some of these habits will certainly last because I *never* want to go back to where I was when I was at my lowest.

The most important advice I have for someone who is about to begin to use a heart rate monitor is not to begin if you can't deal with the truth of what you will find and if you are not willing to make changes. Otherwise, you would be better off remaining blissfully ignorant. If you want to make some changes, using a monitor is your best compass for forging ahead. This will give you indisputable evidence about how you are doing, which changes you have to make, and whether or not the changes are making an impact.

If you are feeling impatient right now, already have a heart rate monitor, are not that fond of theory, and are itching to get started, then you can go straight to the practical section of this book on page 75 and begin working. You can certainly return to the theoretical section of this book when you feel the need to do so. But if what I have presented so far is completely unfamiliar to you, then it may be worth investing a couple of hours becoming acquainted with some of the theoretical knowledge that I think is necessary to get the most out of this book.

THE
THEORY

Just as you are required to take a theoretical course before you are allowed to drive on the road, it is necessary to acquire some theoretical knowledge to benefit fully from the practical sections in this book. In the following pages you are going to learn about how our bodies and brains developed over millions of years and why our current lifestyles are wearing us down and making us ill. You will learn about the immune system and its connection to heart rate variability, which we are going to measure. I can promise you that, once you have absorbed the information here, you will know more about this aspect of preventative health than most doctors.

The brain

We are all fortunate to be equipped with the known universe's most advanced product: the human brain. Human beings share a common ancestor with the fruit fly dating from 800 million years ago and with a chimpanzee six million years ago. We bear with us an evolutionary legacy in which factors that affected fruit flies and chimpanzees also impact us.

About 300,000 years ago we became the species Homo Sapiens, which means *wise human* in Latin. Evolution has unfolded as if it had been constructed with one brick on top of another. Every time something was found to work, it was kept and built upon. That's why we still share 60% of our genes with the fruit fly and 98.9% with chimpanzees.

Our nervous system therefore not only contains advanced human brain cells, but also has many foundational functions that were developed hundreds of millions of years ago and which we still share with everything that lives (and not only vertebrates). Many of these ancient functions of ours were useful for our ancestors while they lived in accordance with nature. However, because we have long since adapted to completely different surroundings and live at a different tempo, they can create problems for us.

For the sake of simplicity, it is often useful to divide our complex brain into three main parts: the reptilian, mammalian, and human (comprising the cerebral cortex and frontal lobe) brains. This is a gross simplification so I will enclose these terms in quotation marks to emphasise this. These main parts of the brain have developed over millions of years through a complicated interaction with one another such that our reptilian brain is much more advanced than a lizard's and our feelings are much more complex than a rat's. However, this simplification is useful when we try to

23

understand ourselves. I like to think of the brain as a two-storey house that has a cellar. The cellar and the ground floor comprise the physiological part of the brain and the first storey represents the psychological.

The 'reptilian brain' is the darkest one in the illustration, and it forms the basement foundation in our nervous system. It consists of the brainstem, the cerebellum, and the spinal cord, including its nerve fibres which spread out to all the organs in the body. This part of the brain regulates the body's automatic functions such as the heartbeat, breathing, alertness, digestion, and stress level. The sympathetic and parasympathetic nerve fibres issue out from the reptilian brain. It reacts to signs of danger instinctively in order to trigger a mobilisation of energy and it reads the cues that then allow the body to rest and recover. This is the brain's on-off switch. It regulates the functionality in the body's many organs, and these functions are the ones that keep all vertebrates alive. To me, the word *instinct* describes this part of the brain. The *reticular* activating system is found here. It controls the subconscious part of our attention, the one that notices the cyclist that suddenly appears in our peripheral vision before we have consciously done it ourselves.

The 'mammalian brain' forms the nervous system's ground floor. Its development benefitted from the asteroid that wiped out the dinosaurs that were so dominant 65 million years ago; we are all descended from the small mammals and primates who survived. This is due to their superior ability to work together in packs and take care of their offspring. It is precisely this mammalian brain, or *the limbic system* as it is also known, that makes sure that this interaction among members of a herd takes place. It is here that the secretion of hormones is governed, which bind us together and reward our ability to cooperate, as well as fostering our commitment to survive, reproduce, and avoid danger. Our feelings originate from this part of the brain.

Our feelings are to a great degree coloured by the hormones which are related to our survival, such as oxytocin, serotonin, dopamine, adrenaline, and cortisol. In common with other mammals, these bind us together so that we collaborate within a productive hierarchy. We are rewarded with positive feelings when we interact with others. In evolutionary terms, this improves our chances of survival. Roughly put, we can say that dopamine drives us towards an expected reward, serotonin is let into our system when we succeed, and oxytocin is released when we take part in good relationships. We experience discomfort when we are threatened or find ourselves in situations which lower our chances for survival. Cortisol is a stress hormone that mobilises us so we are able to get out of threatening situations in time while adrenaline is like a turbo-charged engine that amplifies the energy present in both positive and negative feelings. I reckon that *intuition* is a word that could be used to describe the functioning of this part of the brain. Intuition is like a shortcut to our collected emotional experience.

And then finally we come to the '**human brain**', or the **cerebral cortex** and its **frontal lobe,** which is the top floor in our nervous system. The cerebral cortex was fully developed about 300,000 years ago, which was around 3.5 billion years after the first cellular life appeared on Earth. We are all descended from this organism in an unbroken reproductive line from then until the present time. As an animal species, we are seemingly unique in our ability to think abstractly, envision what we are not able to immediately see with our eyes, and share it using a highly developed spoken language. In this advanced part of the brain, our thoughts buzz and whirr with plans about the future, reminiscing about the past, and pondering over future tasks. The cerebral cortex has enabled us to invent written language so that my thoughts can be expressed here in words which you can then read and reflect upon. The frontal lobe supplies us with the imagination to envision buildings, the educational system, incandescent lamps, computers, and reality TV series, while providing for the creativity, organisation, and engineering needed to produce them. I think *intellect* is a word that can be used to label this part of the brain. Psychological therapy addresses this portion of our brains.

My main point here is to differentiate between the psychological part of the brain and the physiological. We often place greater value on what we might be able to accomplish by treating the psychological part of the brain – and end up undervaluing the potential that exists in treating the physiological part. Although we have a top floor to be proud of and impressed by, this part of the brain is also dependent upon having a solid foundation or cellar. And it is this very lowest and most primitive level of the brain, the autonomic, self-regulating nervous system, that provides the main focus of this book. It is our inner, living fossil that we all carry with us wherever we go. This wordless part of the brain is the foundation for our physiology which makes sure the body's basic functions keep operating. Nerve signals and hormones that are issued from the reptilian brain regulate the activity in all the body's organs. However, contrary to the strong emphasis placed on noticing the imbalance in our thoughts (which occur in our frontal lobes) and our feelings (which are triggered in our mammalian brains), we direct little attention towards what is going on when our autonomic nervous systems are out of balance. When the walls in the first floor tremble, we tend to investigate the immediate surroundings to find the cause. And rightly – thoughts residing in the intellectual part of the brain can cause harm to us as well as emotional discomfort originating in the mammalian brain. However, the reason why the walls are shaking can just as easily be due to weaknesses in the foundation. The central project of this book is to find and repair these weaknesses, that is, the imbalances in the autonomic nervous system. From my experience, this is often where our problems originate.

Trine Helen (50)

As someone who has ME/CFS, a fitness tracker is a good aid for me at work for adjusting my level of activity. I have actively monitored my heart rate for several years, eventually doing it with Garmin's Body Battery to measure my stress. It helps me to improve my health gradually. I have also discovered the impact that temperature has on my body. If I am too warm, my heart rate and stress data leap up. If I remain cool, my stress level settles down quite a bit. Breathing exercises and cold showers lasting one or two minutes also reduce stress. Drinking alcohol results in a lot of stress. Too much food or food I can't really tolerate, sweets, and late meals result in a lot of stress that lingers for hours afterwards, and this negatively affects the quality of my sleep. The most surprising measurement I have noticed was when I gave a lecture to a class at an upper secondary school. While I was talking, the monitor showed a very low stress reading the entire time.

The autonomic nervous system

The autonomic nervous system is well-hidden both in our bodies and from common knowledge. If the term is unknown to you, be comforted by the fact that you are not alone. I've been studying this subject for four or five years, and when I mention it, most people say, 'What's that?!' Even doctors and other healthcare workers express surprise when I explain that the heartbeat variability that I measure with my gadgets is able to reveal the state of our autonomic nervous system. The nervous system lies deep inside our bodies and does its job unnoticed so long as things are going well. In fact, our bodies seem to suppress signals from the autonomic nervous system so as not to disturb our attention on external sensory impressions.

I like to compare the autonomic nervous system to the drivetrain in a car which comprises the axles, valves, gearbox, and suspension. It consists of everything that is hidden under the bonnet and that rarely gives us problems. But if we fail to change the oil, or let the tyres wear thin, or neglect the gearbox, the car will break down and even the most advanced electronics system will be of no use. So it is with the autonomic nervous system, which provides the driving force in our body. As long as it gets enough sleep, rest, exercise, and good food, it can work smoothly until we get old. But in these hectic times, the nervous system is often stretched beyond capacity.

I've already mentioned that the autonomic nervous system consists of two parts that work in tandem to create equilibrium in the body: the *sympathetic* and *parasympathetic* systems. The sympathetic system is like an 'accelerator' or 'on button'. The parasympathetic system is like a 'brake' or 'off button'.

The sympathetic nervous system activates stress and mobilises us into action. It increases the heart rate, slows digestion, makes us less sleepy, dilates the pupils, and increases alertness. It releases glucose and hormones that prepare us for flight from something frightening, or to hunt something desirable. Maintenance work in the body is put on hold, so that our energy can be directed towards the activity that ensures our immediate survival. The sympathetic nerve signals are sent from the brain, through the spinal cord, and through the nerve fibres out to all the body's organs.

The autonomic nervous system developed when our ancestors lived under the ever-present threat of attack from wild animals. What threatens most of us now is our frenzied lifestyle. If we are constantly in the sympathetic mode – in an activated or mobilised mode – we become exhausted. The body, brain, and immune system fall prey to inflammation, which brings with it troubling symptoms that reduce our quality of life. Worse still, inflammation creates fertile ground for various chronic and fatal diseases.

To avoid this disease-inducing state, the autonomic nervous system calls upon the *parasympathetic* system. Its job is to allow both the body and mind to recover and de-stress and thus the restoration of energy after effort. When the situation allows, the parasympathetic nervous system clocks in. We can rest, our muscles are repaired, digestion is prioritised, the immune system has a chance to get to work, we fall asleep more easily, and the brain is cleared of waste substances produced from the day's thinking.

The brain issues parasympathetic signals to all our body's organs via the *vagus nerve*. The word *vagus* has the same root as vagabond, and with good reason. This wandering nerve originates in the brainstem, and travels through the body to all our internal organs, giving out signals that mitigate the stress activated by the sympathetic nervous system in these same organs.

The sympathetic nervous system is permanently activated – as though the accelerator were always on – while the parasympathetic nervous system is like a brake we must actively engage. Or, more precisely, prepare the body to engage. While you can whip yourself into action, you cannot compel restitution. You can only seek calm and allow recovery to occur.

This on-off function in the two divisions of the nervous system exists in most organisms. And if we want to promote health, we would do well to attend to this legacy. To function at our best, we must be able to mobilise our forces when we need to, while ensuring adequate recovery. It is this balance that heart rate monitors can help us to find.

The autonomic nervous system

You have probably heard of the automatic responses to threat: *fight, flight,* or *freeze.* The sympathetic nervous system is responsible for activating these responses. It is what saved us on the savannah from animals that wanted to eat us, or tribes that wanted to kill us. It is what helps us escape unwanted situations. But the sympathetic nervous system is also activated by pleasure responses, such as when we are hunting or playing. It mobilises us towards things we need and desire, which was, of course, equally important to our survival. So even when an activity is exciting, fun, or meaningful, it can also drain the body's battery – something you will learn more about later.

The parasympathetic nervous system institutes recovery and rest after we have been in the fear zone or the pleasure zone. In fact, our physiology evolved for us to spend most of the day in this relaxed condition, not the opposite, as we so often do nowadays. The time we devote to the slow recovery process is simply too short when we spend so much of the day in sympathetic mode, that is activated, mobilised, or 'switched on'.

To gain control of the balance between these two systems is to acknowledge the animal in us. We are not merely human. We are human animals. And if we overlook the animal in ourselves, we also become less human; ultimately, we have less energy to utilise our advanced brains.

Using heart rate monitors as our compass, we are about to go on an expedition into the world of our autonomic nervous system.

But first, we need to equip ourselves with more knowledge.

Hanne (52)
I always believed I grew tired by being around people and have consequently withdrawn myself from certain situations and spent a lot of time alone. So, it came as a big surprise to me when I began monitoring the Body Battery. It showed that I am in fact charging my batteries to a greater degree when I am spending time with close friends than when I am alone. Knowing this has enabled me to change my way of thinking. Spending time with other people gives me greater joy today than it did before.

The drawbacks of
the mammalian brain

In the context of evolution, we parted ways with mice 75 million years ago, but we still use them to stand in for our physiology in medical research. That says something about how old our operating systems are. So, although the reptilian brain is the main subject of this book, it may be helpful to have a quick look at how the mammalian brain, or the limbic system, affects us.

The hormones that are regulated from this part of the brain – dopamine, serotonin, and oxytocin – comprise the main drivers behind our motivation to collaborate with others to get things done. If we block the release of dopamine in animal testing, a mammal will lose its motivation even for such an essential activity as eating. And if the release of oxytocin is blocked, then a mother will neglect her offspring. Cortisol troubles us when our brains interpret something we experience as being a threat to our survival, such as, for example, when the lives of other people appear better than ours do on Facebook. These ones are called 'emotional hormones' because they colour and shape our moods.

It may be worth our while to know something about these hormones and pheromones so that we can sit back and relax when this ancient, non-verbal part of the brain begins to affect us. These hormones are not exactly designed for thriving in a modern society; they are more suited for helping our ancestors survive in Africa millions of years ago.

There are three mammalian brain-related pitfalls that are of significance for determining and shaping the mood we are in.

The first pitfall: comparing yourself to other people. Mammalian survival is closely connected to our intense striving to compare ourselves to others. We get a serotonin kick when we feel that we are better than those we compare ourselves to and a charge of cortisol when it feels like the opposite. One consequence of this is that we avoid fighting those who are stronger than we are. We can more readily ensure our survival by adapting and finding our place in certain hierarchies. Apes are the most interested in those higher up the social structure – particularly in their love lives and conflicts – as for them it is a matter of survival. We only need to look at an online news publication to see that we humans are engrossed with the same things. When we are bombarded with the lives of the powerful and the seemingly successful on every channel and platform, we feel inferior and insignificant. We compare our hidden, messy feelings about ourselves with the visible, polished surfaces of other people. Just relax, take a deep breath, and let it go when these feelings appear, acknowledging that they are the remnants of an ancient survival mechanism. Instead, turn to look for something that brings you pleasure and joy!

The second pitfall: placing too much attention on what is negative. Focusing on what is negative is another attribute that has strengthened our ability to survive. Those of our ancestors who were alert to threats fared better than the ones who just smelled the flowers and patted their bellies contentedly. The problem with this lies in how it pans out in our modern age: we get just as upset by a negative comment on social media as our ancestors did by hearing a lion roar nearby. The hypothalamus, an almond-sized gland located in the mammalian brain which controls these types of reactions, struggles to differentiate between significant and insignificant threats. In other words, the hypothalamus is utterly overwhelmed when the time comes to handle all the impressions coming in from the frontal lobe. Humans have been designed to put their attention on what they lack or appears to be a threat rather than focus on what they have or what brings them happiness. Try to compensate for this inherent characteristic of ours by being grateful for all you do have in your life and think about how *difficult* life would be if you did *not* have it.

The third pitfall: our extreme capacity for adaptation. Our third ability, which was and still is useful but torments us all the same, is our wide-ranging ability to adapt and adjust ourselves to our surroundings. We take new situations for granted instantly. All the incredible things around us are taken as a matter of course and we become blasé. We quickly become accustomed to the new gadgets or clothing we purchase and begin looking around for something new or better. Instead, try looking at the world around you from the viewpoint of an alien from another planet, a great-great-grandmother coming back to visit, or a child. Notice the small things that are in fact great in significance once we truly see them.

We should send a thank you to our ancestors, who were survivors, because they were able to pass on their genes to us. At the same time, we can learn to relax, let loose a little, smile and tell ourselves that this mental inheritance of ours is something we need about as much as we need axes and spears. That is, if we hope to have peace of mind and joy enter our lives.

Recommended reading
I, Mammal: How to Make Peace with the Animal Urge for Social Power by Loretta G. Breuning
Behave: The Biology of Humans at Our Best and Worst by Robert Sapolsky

Gunhild (46)
I have learnt to not eat too often. Whole, plant-based food has little impact on stress and ultra-processed foods have a greater one. It's the same with alcohol; one unit is OK. Bathing in the sea or taking a cold shower for two or three minutes allows me to charge for about two hours afterwards. Breathing exercises and meditations are worth their weight in gold. Becoming aware of being present works well. When I am in a state of flow, even in a work situation, I am charging. Mental stress is burdensome, such as when I am rushing to get something done or feel like I should have been somewhere else. Scheduling breaks for active rest during the day results in a better quality of sleep at night.

The immune system

Now that we have looked inside our body, it is time to turn our gaze towards what I call the 'disease landscape' that is leaving its mark on our society. Over the course of the last 150 years, we have made the natural landscape around us almost unrecognisable by building cities, roads, dams, and agricultural areas. Half of the Earth's habitable areas are now being used for agriculture. Biodiversity is plummeting. The seas have been nearly emptied of fish and are being used as a rubbish bin. The planet is boiling over with greenhouse gasses. In the same way, the disease landscape has also become unrecognisable. We have shifted from diseases of poverty to diseases of wealth. Infectious diseases have been replaced by inflammatory diseases. And it seems to be just as difficult to save our minds and bodies from the poisonous lifestyle that characterises the age we live in, as it is to reverse the negative developments that have taken place in nature in order to save the planet and the oceans. To understand certain connections between lifestyle diseases and heart rate variability, which we can measure on our own, we need to better familiarise ourselves with our immune system and the diseases themselves. Many people talk about the necessity of having a strong immune system. However, it is more precise to say that we need a *balanced* immune system, one that attacks the right intruders when it is supposed to and does not turn on its own cells when it is not. For this to happen, our stress needs to be balanced well. This is the goal of the stages that will be presented later in this book. If our level of stress grows too high, we enter a state of chronic inflammation.

My simplified picture of our immune system in such a state is as follows: if, over a long period of time, a person is continuously subjected to stress without getting sufficient rest, their immune system starts to function as if it consists of new military recruits who, hyper-alert, suddenly jump up and shoot wildly in all directions, causing all sorts of trouble. At the same time, the amount and intensity of the noise they make mean that the more precise, experienced, and better equipped officers of the immune system put their hands over their ears and close their eyes. The result can be outbreaks of autoimmune diseases as well as deficiencies in the body's defence against cell damage, uncontrolled cell growth such as cancers, or a reduced capacity to fight off infections.

This is essentially all the information you need to make use of the measures presented in this book. However, if you have the time and patience to absorb more complicated, scientific knowledge, then please do read on!

THE TWO-PART IMMUNE SYSTEM

The immune system is highly advanced and consists of two main parts: the *innate* and the *adaptive* immune systems. Developed throughout evolution, these natural forces within ourselves are our best warriors against disease. The primitive innate immune system first appeared billions of years ago in single-celled lifeforms, which were amoebas. The adaptive immune system emerged 500 million years ago in jawed fish, and it was even further perfected for doing this work. Both parts are based on immune cells that are formed in our bone marrow and they are both dependent on a good stress balance. The innate immune system consists of, among other things, immune cells that are present in our tissues, especially near the skin and mucous membranes that are exposed to the outside world, such as, for example, in the gastrointestinal tract and in the lungs. If there is a suspicious intruder, they report it quickly, and warn the adaptive immune system. The innate immune system's cells respond quickly. However, they are also imprecise and have a poor memory. When the same enemy attacks again, they start all over again from scratch.

The adaptive immune system consists of B- and T-cells. It may take several days for these cells to be activated to make an effort, but in return they are precise, and they do not forget details about the germs they have battled before. This is beneficial for us when an intruder enters from outside our bodies. However, with regard to autoimmune diseases, their efficiency and long-term memory can work against us when they encounter a genuinely benign threat originating from within our body.

CLOSE INTEGRATION WITH THE BRAIN

The immune system is closely integrated with the functioning of the brain. This system is not a passive one that waits until damage has been done before it jumps into action. Instead it listens to the brain and is mobilised when certain states of mind are present, which in the Stone Age indicated that there existed an increased risk of imminent harm, such as loneliness, stress, frustration, fear, bitterness, anger, and being worried. Our thoughts, feelings, and moods literally communicate with the immune system in real time and regulate the functioning of the immune cells. The reason that these emotional states continue to affect us is because the basic principles of our immune systems have remained unchanged for the last 500 million years. This is something we share with other jawed vertebrates.

A SELF-REGULATING SYSTEM

When an immune response has begun, much of the task of the immune system comes down to regulating itself so that a particular response is sufficiently strong and will last long enough. There is, among others, a group of regulatory cells called, T-reg cells. Their job is to slow down other immune cells. In instances of a chronic state of stress, these cells fail to work, and this can lead to the appearance of an illness.

Anne-Lise (60)
I am able to have control over my fatigue on a day-to-day basis. When I had to deal with some additional stress due to a long-standing conflict with my neighbour, it all went south, and I was left with a lot of negative stress. After one meeting with the neighbour, my energy level plummeted and I was unable to recharge. It was difficult to turn things around. The watch helped me handle the situation better than I had done in the past. I had to rest quite a bit in order to recover.

THE IMPACT OF STRESS

When we are feeling stressed our immune cells excrete *cytokines*, and these cause inflammation. Historically, this has been relevant to short-term stress-inducing situations followed by restitution. If the stress persists, however, a state marked by chronic, disease-causing inflammation ensues. This leads to damage being done to our tissues and increases the risk of organ failure, a propensity towards infection, and the development of cancer and autoimmune diseases.

When energy is expended while dealing with stress, we have less of it available for the immune system. One example of this is when the stress resulting from a sleepless night reduces the activity of vital *natural killer cells* by 70%. Natural killer cells are a type of lymphocyte cell similar to B- and T-cells, which monitor and kill cancer cells and virus-infected cells in particular. People who sleep six hours or less a night have four times the risk of catching a cold than those who sleep for seven hours or more. These cells are an important weapon against cancer, and for those who sleep poorly at night, the risk of cancer in fact doubles.

The cells in the immune system are among those in the body that regenerate the quickest. The lifespan of many immune cells is only 100 days. Our defence capabilities are dependent upon the quality of the 'conscripts' that are available to serve at any given time. This is both positive and negative. It means that if you have taken great steps forward to improve your immune system, then it may not take long before your health reaps the benefits. On the other hand, going through a very stressful period can contribute to bringing your immune system to its knees in a relatively short amount of time, and so to an increased risk of serious illness.

Fortunately, we can monitor the state of our immune systems by measuring our heart rate variability.

According to immunologist Jenna Macciochi:

'HRV is an excellent estimator of your overall immune health. In a low-HRV state, your system is working overtime to maintain the processes required for physiological homeostasis. As a result, your body is less capable of adapting to acute stressors. Suppression of your HRV relative to your baseline is a sign of under-recovery and greater susceptibility to illness. It can even indicate the early stages of infection or inflammation before you have symptoms. This is because HRV is very sensitive to inflammatory pathways – including changes driven by the innate immune system – as it ramps up to combat runaway viral replication. Often, your morning HRV will change abruptly and surprisingly, signalling the onset of illness. HRV is easily trackable using wearable devices and free smartphone apps.'

Recommended reading
Immunity: The Science of Staying Well by Dr Jenna Macciochi

Anita (58)
The data shows that I actually had a lot of stress in my body even when I thought I was relaxing. I was surprised to see that what you eat, your amount of activity, and drinking alcohol have such a big effect on stress levels. Thanks to what I have learnt about HRV, stress, the Body Battery, and what affects all of these, I am well on my way to a full recovery. I've got a tool that helps me to regulate and balance my energy so that I can avoid experiencing a big crash. Now, most often I am able to stop a crash in time.

This tool helps me to understand, balance, and regulate the silent part of my body that we aren't aware of until it is too late and shouts: 'I'm done! Stop!' I think that what I have learnt will help me to have a full recovery of my health and prevent a relapse and being burnt out again.

For a while I felt like I was just existing, so THANK YOU SO MUCH for giving me the opportunity to participate in this project and teaching me to use a tool that has helped me get my life back.

From infection to inflammation

In 1999 I was doing my residency at Nordland Hospital in Bodø, Norway. After receiving an education in which we became familiar with the most exceptional instances of disease at Oslo University Hospital, I went out into the field to encounter what makes up the more common, everyday ones that we face. At that time, we did not have digital medical record files. So, we were handed a file that just from its volume and weight alone told us a great deal about the patient before we had even shaken hands. You could measure the illness-induced stress they were living with in kilograms just from weighing the paper files. I remember one day being at the pulmonary department when it hit me: 'How was it possible for one person to accumulate so many different diseases in their entire body?'

I met patients who had to gulp down 15 to 20 different medicinal concoctions a day, each one with its own menu of side effects that were impossible to keep track of. At medical school we had learnt about each individual disease in isolation, but no one had told us about how a profusion of them could wind up accumulating in groups of vulnerable people. The basic contents in a pill organiser usually contained two or three different blood pressure medications, anticoagulants, two or three different diabetes medications, cholesterol-lowering medication, medication for having too much stomach acid, prostate medication, anti-inflammatory medication, metabolic medication, antidepressants, and asthma medication.

What perhaps made it especially difficult when looking for a common denominator among the various diseases was the number of specialists involved with each patient. Lung specialists treated them for asthma, endocrinologists for metabolism, gynaecologists for polycystic ovary syndrome, heart specialists for atrial fibrillation, surgeons for ulcerative colitis, urologists for prostate problems, psychiatrists for depression, gastroenterologists for gastritis, rheumatologists for arthritis, neurologists for polyneuropathy, oncologists for breast cancer, and ophthalmologists treated for Sjögren's syndrome. I could continue like this *ad absurdum*. Perhaps the problem was that nobody was looking for a common denominator. Everyone dealt with their part of the patient and none of them, and certainly not their GP, was instructed to look for what linked all the diseases together during their 15-minute consultation. A GP has more than enough to do with administering all the discharge summaries and referrals and the lists of medications, which are often altered after each appointment with a specialist. I was to meet many of these people who had diagnoses and treatments in multiple illnesses in the years that followed.

Today, we know something that we did not know at the time: a general, chronic inflammatory state provides the basis for many of the aforementioned diseases whether they are mental or physical. According to psychiatrist and doctor Jeffrey Rediger at Harvard Medical School, only 5–10% of diseases have arisen by chance or can be due to the genes we inherit. In 90–95% of all instances of disease, our modern, inflammation-causing lifestyle is the common factor among them. Rediger points out that as soon as this lifestyle starts to incorporate the activities and rhythm of the life we were evolutionarily developed to live, and begins to resemble it to a greater degree, then, in many cases, we will be able to drop many of these medications one by one. Fortunately, the level of the body's inflammatory state can be revealed in the heart rate variability since the sympathetic nervous system is activated by inflammation.

Therese (42)
Almost everything I do, when I'm not sleeping, creates a stress response in my body. This applies to everything from showering, eating, and talking on the phone to surfing on the web and gardening. When I began to realise this, I became more careful with what I spent my time and energy on.

The disease landscape in the Western world has changed radically during the last few decades. Our bodies are still in an inflamed condition. However, from being dominated by infectious diseases such as tuberculosis, pneumonia, diphtheria, and diarrhoea, which we gradually have become good at avoiding or curing through hygiene, vaccines, and antibiotics, the overall range of illnesses now consists predominantly of inflammatory diseases such as heart disease, cancer, diabetes, chronic pulmonary disease, stroke, dementia, and kidney diseases. We do not have equally effective medications for these diseases.

Many people mix up the terms *infection* and *inflammation*. Due to evolution, the immune system is adapted to attack external enemies, such as bacteria in wounds, germs from other people or domesticated animals, and to protect us from spoiled food and drink. The body's immune cells then expel inflammatory substances, which quickly activate the immune system to neutralise the intruder quickly and effectively. When the effects of the infection have settled down, the attack is supposed to be called off. And now that we have been able to ward off such attacks through the help of effective vaccines, good hygiene, food safety, and clean water – and in addition have effective antibiotics to combat any attacks that should nevertheless arise – you would think we would be able to live an inflammation-free life to a greater extent than we do now. But this is not the case. The inflammation diseases that are now ravaging the bodies of many of us are triggered by our modern lifestyle. Our immune system has millions of years of experience handling diseases caused by injuries, bacteria, parasites, viruses, and hunger, but hardly any for fighting against our present lifestyle diseases.

The external threats, which previously caused many instances of *infection*, have been replaced by internal ones, which often lead to *inflammation*. Inflammatory substances – cytokines – are also secreted when we sleep too little, rest too rarely, move insufficiently, eat too much ultra-processed food, weigh too much, and become stressed out too often. This state results in a continuous, low-grade inflammatory condition that over time wears down our bodies and leads to the proliferation of a range of lifestyle diseases that are predominant in today's disease landscape. As well as creating poor conditions for the regulation of immune cells, in the absence of external enemies, the firepower of the immune system turns on our own bodies, resulting in the devasting effects of 'friendly fire' – autoimmune diseases such as arthritis, allergies, asthma, multiple sclerosis, psoriasis, and Crohn's disease, as well as a long list of others.

These internally triggered inflammatory diseases have one advantage: we can get some control over them through living a healthy lifestyle. In the past, people had less control over infectious diseases. But we already have the means for healing these inflammatory-based illnesses within us, namely the immune system. However, if it is going to work optimally, we have to activate the parasympathetic nervous system in its recovery mode in our physiology.

The lifestyle that offers our bodies opportunities to promote good health resembles the one that has been dominant throughout evolution. It features regular exercise, natural food, sufficient sleep, fasting, and periods of stress that build and enhance mental and physical strength and resilience.

Synnøve (38)
I have a lot of stress in my everyday life. Seeing this in summary form every day makes me more aware that I have to schedule and set aside some quiet periods for myself.

Cortisol is the hormone that regulates our immune responses. In an acute, stressful situation cortisol effectively distributes resources to the places where they need to go. Problems arise when we are in a chronic inflammatory state. In such an instance, the tissues will have become acclimatised to a higher, continuous level of cortisol and the ability of the immune system to regulate its response will deteriorate. The cells in the immune system cease to listen. They become confused, frantic, and disorganised. These mutinous forces have thus revolted from the army and no longer follow the orders of 'General Cortisol'. They plunder and pillage the body's tissues at their own discretion.

Low-grade, chronic stress is a cause of disease all on its own. In addition, at my practice I have often sensed that outbreaks of life-threatening diseases such as cancer and heart disease occur when people who already have a lot of stress in their lives encounter an acute situation which tips the balance. In addition, several studies have indicated that about 80% of those people who develop autoimmune diseases have reported experiencing an instance of extraordinary and unexpected emotional stress entering their lives just before the first symptoms start. I would be interested to find out the extent to which inflammatory and infectious diseases occur after people begin divorce proceedings, deal with work issues, undergo a criminal investigation, or go through the illness or death of close family members.

One aspect related to inflammation that is perhaps surprising is that symptoms of depression can arise due to it, which is called *sickness behaviour*. Inflammatory diseases create the same symptoms as infectious diseases: we become lethargic and are less active, withdraw ourselves from social interaction, and think negative thoughts. British psychiatrist and professor Edward Bullmore, the author of the book *The Inflamed Mind*, says:

'These days it is difficult to think of a disease that isn't caused or complicated by inflammation or auto-immunity. And it is equally difficult to think of a disease that isn't associated with depression, fatigue, anxiety, or some other mental symptom.'

The good, and at the same time bad, news is that the best medications for us are in fact free, effective, and easily available to us: good sleep, sufficient exercise, good stress management, rest, participation in meaningful activities, healthy food, being hydrated, socialising with others, being exposed to the cold such as in showers, breathing exercises, and being present and attentive in the moment. All of this provides the body's immune system with the conditions it needs to do the job it does best and has taken millions of years to learn – keeping us healthy.

However, precisely because these medications are free, no one is going to promote them to you. The pharmaceutical industry and much of the healthcare sector have everything to gain from people barely hanging on while their immune systems weaken to the point where a lot of resources have to be used diagnosing and treating the resulting illness. And because the treatments are often ineffective, many patients end up needing that help for the rest of their lives.

Patients have to be told that an alternative to drugs actually exists, one whose positive effect has been proven. By studying heart rate variability, we can discover the degree of inflammation in our bodies. The connection between the two is most likely as follows: a persistently stressed, overactive autonomic nervous system leads to chronic inflammation in the body and, thus, the immune system functions poorly. Consequently, a vicious circle begins: the defectively functioning immune system increases the risk of disease, which in its turn intensifies the burden put on the autonomic nervous system. If your heart rate variability (the HRV value) is low, then this is one of several possible reasons for it.

Recommended reading
Cured: The Power of Our Immune System and the Mind-Body Connection by Dr Jeff Rediger
The Inflamed Mind: A Radical New Approach to Depression by Edward Bullmore

Ellen (58)
After undergoing a caesarean section 25 years ago, my body has more or less been in a state of sympathetic stress ever since. So, I have struggled with sleep disorders and everything that often accompanies them, such as being burnt out, depression, digestive disorders, ME/CFS, anxiety, and migraines. Consequently, I am extremely sensitive to stress. EVERYTHING stresses me out and the monitors show that I have to do something actively for my body to enter into a parasympathetic state.

Diseases you can prevent

Which diseases are triggered by inflammation?

Many people believe that there is a distinction between lifestyle diseases and other diseases. However, there are hardly any diseases that are not triggered or influenced by one's lifestyle. Put simply, our lifestyle affects our immune systems, and our immune systems have an impact on both our risk of contracting a disease and our ability to recover from it. Even in the case of cancer, eight of the ten most common forms will appear in the organs in which the flow of blood has been reduced due to stress.

When I studied medicine in the 1990s, it was hardly mentioned that a person could independently implement measures to improve their health. On the contrary, we got the impression that diseases were hereditary and, in a way, unavoidable, or that people were afflicted by them randomly and that therefore those people were simply unfortunate – which is nearly as unavoidable. Smoking, of course, was an exception to this. In the 1970s, people finally began to realise and understand the damaging effects of nicotine. But this wasn't always the case in every instance – during this same decade, my own mother was advised by her doctor to use smoking as a slimming aid. That says a little about how long it can take for some rather obvious facts to make their way into a curriculum.

What I remember from my time at medical school is that knowledge trickled from deadly serious, arrogant professors and bone-dry, door-stopper-sized books down to us impressionable students who were quite eager to learn and absorb it. This was a time before the internet was as interactive and as widespread as it is today. Now, knowledge spreads quickly, and new scientific discoveries can just as easily be found by young, innovative, enthusiastic people as they can by professors. Adventurer Dan Buettner exemplifies this type of person. He came up with the simple idea of looking for common features in the lifestyles of the people in the areas in the world where they have the longest lifespans.

These areas, called *Blue Zones*, turned out to have some interesting key lifestyle habits in common. The inhabitants were regularly active, ate moderately, were slim, and enjoyed a mainly plant-based diet. They prioritised having enough time for proper sleep and rest as well as spending time with family and at other social gatherings. They thought that their everyday lives had meaning and purpose. And they did not just live longer – Buettner also noted that they were happier and healthier. Perhaps these solutions were too simple for a prestige-orientated doctor to search for and find.

The medical truths of the previous century are increasingly losing their relevance. Several new research findings have shaken things up: the lifestyle we lead dictates the state of our health to an extent that would have seemed inconceivable to a doctor in the last millennium. Examples of new research findings and discoveries include epigenetics (how our behaviour and environment can cause changes that affect the way genes work), the plasticity of the brain (how the brain can be shaped by experiences), telomeres (the protective ends of chromosomes – they show that our lifestyle influences molecules that protect our genetic material), the impact on the body of the gut's microbiota (diversity of bacteria in the gut), the connection between exercise and mental health, the significance of inflammation and insulin resistance (a state where the insulin-driven transfer of glucose to the cells is reduced, which affects access to energy and thus the function of all the body's cells), and the importance of the circadian rhythm. A couple of hours browsing through videos on these subjects on YouTube can teach you more about preventing disease than we had access to as doctors back in the analogue age. The pyramid of knowledge seems to have been turned on its head, and that's a good thing.

I have now worked as a doctor for the length of a whole generation, and it is obvious as well as indisputable to me that the majority of the diseases we suffer from, are medicated for, and die from are preventable. In the defence of doctors from a previous age, it can of course be noted that people's lifestyles were completely different in the past and that they included more exercise, better sleep, more social interaction, fewer environmental toxins as well as a diet in which snacks, quick carbohydrates, and ultra-processed food were less prominent. Most likely, the lifestyles people lived were much more similar for everyone across the board and there were fewer significant differences between those who lived in either a healthy or unhealthy way.

Now, none of us who work as doctors in the 21st century can excuse ourselves by saying we do not have a sufficient general comprehension of the importance of one's lifestyle for their health. Even I have to admit that my own understanding has been lacking and give myself a slap on the wrist for it. Just six or seven years ago I too was not aware of the degree to which we can all influence our health.

Below you will see a brief overview of the diseases that shape and fill my working hours at my practice, as well as generating billions of dollars in revenue for the pharmaceutical and healthcare industries. These industries will hopefully start shaking at their foundations as people gradually become aware of the potential that lies within preventative healthcare. The use of heart rate monitors as well as the optimisation of our autonomic nervous systems and physiology will limit the incidences of disease significantly.

According to studies cited by the Foundations of Heart Rate Variability course at the Elite Academy (academy.elitehrv.com), a connection has been found between heart rate variability and the following diseases:

Heart diseases	Prostate problems
Alzheimer's disease	Anxiety
Cancer	Infertility
Sleep disorders	Digestive issues
Stroke	Erectile dysfunction
High blood pressure	Diabetes
Depression	Autoimmune diseases

Here it must be pointed out that we do not have a full picture of the causal relationships underpinning this connection yet. Does a low heart rate variability cause the onset of the disease, or does the disease manifest itself in a low heart rate variability? The answer to this is most likely due to an interaction between the two within a vicious cycle, or, more precisely, a vicious downward spiral.

Recommended reading
The Blue Zones: Secrets for Living Longer – Lessons From the Healthiest Places on Earth by Dan Buettner
Brain Energy by Christopher Palmer

> **Anette (44)**
> After 16 years working as a neuro reflexologist, it is exciting for me to consider what opportunities we now have for the measurement of treatment outcomes, and how I, by studying the patients' monitors, can help them to improve their health. The outcomes reveal, among other things, an increase in the Body Battery, the amount of sleep they get, the presence of deep sleep, and their HRV. The patients not only feel better, but they also have received a confirmation of how they have felt through their individual, concrete data.

Healthy living in the Stone Age

After reading hundreds of books on the latest discoveries in medicine and psychology, one thing seems obvious to me, and it is that most modern medicine has its roots in the ancient past. The following message is short and sweet: we have to live a little more like our earliest hunter and gatherer ancestors. Their lifestyle, which has been the dominant one during the entirety of the evolution of human beings, save the last couple of thousands of years, can make us healthier. If we were to live closer to this lifestyle, we would get good results on our monitors.

What did the hunters and gatherers do? For the most part, the same things they do today. They sleep when it is dark, hunt, gather, and catch what they need to survive on, rest when they can, are seldom alone, eat natural foods, dance for the fun of it, keep fit, create and make tools, instruments, and jewellery, fast when food is scarce, and continue to play well into old age. However, the tribes that still live this way, such as the Hadza in Tanzania or the Tsimané in Bolivia, have long since been displaced and forced out to areas that have poor living conditions. Despite this, social anthropologists can affirm there are very low incidences of depression, heart disease, and cancer in these tribal communities. The blood vessels of 80-year-old men are as clean as a man aged 50 in the West. However, they are exposed to infections, accidents, and violent deaths, men in particular.

Let's look at some identifiable features of these two lifestyles.

The Stone Age	Modern life
Sufficient sleep	Insufficient sleep
Natural circadian rhythm	Unnatural, disrupted circadian rhythm
Natural food	Ultra-processed food
Time spent outdoors in nature	Time spent indoors, little exposure to nature
Natural movement	Sedentary activity
Plentiful rest	Seldom at rest
Togetherness	Loneliness
Play	Absence of play
Fasting	Eating at all hours
Very little fast-acting carbohydrates (for example, sugar and flour)	Lots of fast-acting carbohydrates
Varied immune-boosting intestinal flora	Homogenous, immune-depleting intestinal flora
Normal body weight	Overweight
Freedom	Lack of freedom
Fear	Anxiety
A lot of exposure to the sun and natural light	Relatively dim light from light bulbs
Dancing	No dancing
Sitting on the floor and rising often	Sitting in chairs and sofas
Rituals	Few rituals
Natural breaks in time	Time-squeeze

Of course, we do not have to return to the savannah or the jungle to restore our health, but if we make certain adjustments in line with the way hunters and gatherers lived in previous times, we can improve our health and increase our well-being. Going from nothing to something is in fact quite a big gain!

If we work against our biology by following the lifestyle outlined in the right-hand column on the previous page, we will ultimately lose. And these losses can be measured in our health and the length of our lifespan. Our goal should be to get our bodies to team up with biology, and not go against it. We do not need to return to nature; we should instead become accustomed to living more naturally.

Recommended reading

The Depression Cure: The Six-Step Programme to Beat Depression Without Drugs by Dr Steve Ilardi

Be More Human: How to Transform Your Lifestyle for Optimum Health, Happiness and Vitality by Tony Riddle

> **Annette (38)**
> I was surprised that being exposed to the cold was critical for the Body Battery staying at a reasonable level. So, it suits me quite well that I have ended up settling on a windy island out in a rural fjord area.

Miracle biometrics:
heart rate variability

There is a tool that can gauge whether our autonomic nervous system is in sympathetic or parasympathetic mode. To measure heart rate variability (HRV), we use the two most important vital functions: our heartbeat and the rhythm of our breath. Our breathing and pulse are the very foundation of life; they are what keep us alive. Was this so obvious that we overlooked it? For me – involved as I am, every day, in more complex laboratory data and experiments – it is almost touching that these two very basic functions might offer the key to measuring the state of our nervous system and our physiology.

But what exactly is heart rate variability, or HRV?

Our pulse rate rises as we inhale and fill our lungs with oxygen and falls as we exhale. This saves the heart a great deal of work since in this phase our lungs have less oxygen to carry over into the red blood cells. The difference in heart rate can be quite large, from 90 beats per minute on inhalation to 60 beats per minute on exhalation. When we consider that the heart beats around 100,000 times a day, this saving is of enormous benefit. This variation in pulse rate – influenced by whether we are breathing in or out – is called *heart rate variability* (*HRV*), and it offers a window into our nervous system.

In the diagram on page 53, you can see two sets of heartbeats. In the top graph, the heart beats steadily like a clock, with an interval of 845 milliseconds between every beat. The distance between each beat is the same whether the subject is inhaling or exhaling; it has low heart rate variability. This happens when we are under physical or mental stress, that is when the autonomic nervous system is *sympathetically* activated.

This can happen when we exercise, or feel anxious during an important presentation, or nervous before a date or are generally stressed. The pulse then rises, and the nervous system goes into sympathetic mode because it registers that we need extra energy to undertake the task it assumes we are facing. The heart then omits to slow down on exhalation, working instead to ensure an increased supply of oxygen to the muscles and the brain, even if this means 'wasting' some energy. In other words, low heart rate variability indicates that you have a high level of stress.

On the bottom graph you will see that the interval between each heart-beat varies from 732 to 845 milliseconds. This occurs when we are in resting mode and the body is in recovery, i.e. when the autonomic nervous system is *parasympathetically* activated. For example, when we sleep or read, or feel a sense of well-being and peace. If your heart rate variability is high, this reflects a low stress level.

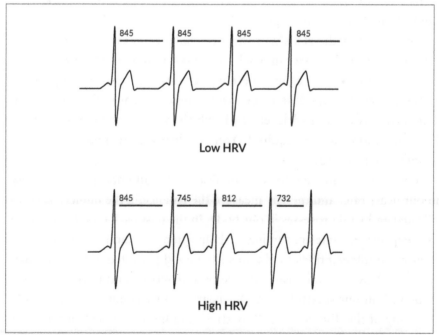

Low HRV

High HRV

Example of heart rhythm and variation in heart rate. A chronic low heart rate variability is negative for one's health (top), a high variability is favourable (bottom).

As we know, the heart beats on its own without any intervention from us. Of course, we can purposely think about something scary and feel our pulse rise, then focus our thoughts on a calm memory and feel it drop again. But in general, the regulation of our heart's rhythm takes place beneath our radar, because the heart receives its orders from the autonomous nervous system. The sympathetic system sends signals so that the heart rate increases, and the parasympathetic system sends mitigating signals, which lower the heart rate. If we were to cut the parasympathetic nerve pathway to our heart, our resting heart rate would be approximately 120 beats per minute, in contrast to the normal 50 to 80. In other words, we can say that our resting heart rate is a measure of how effectively our body can access the parasympathetic nervous system, at any given time.

Breathing is an autonomous, unconscious function, which we can nonetheless control consciously if we choose. We might say that breath is a link by which we can influence the autonomous nervous system. We cannot decide to increase or decrease our pulse, digestion or direct the flow of blood from one organ to another, but we can decide the speed at which we breathe. This will affect the balance in the nervous system. By breathing slowly, we can 'trick' the nervous system into interpreting our environment as calm, thereby activating the parasympathetic system. If we breathe faster, the sympathetic system will be activated. This gives us a 'control lever' with which we can regulate our stress levels up and down as required. You will learn more about this in the chapter on active rest.

With a heart rate monitor we can observe this all-important variability in our heart rate, and thereby measure the balance in the numerous complicated and vital processes in our body. In the past we would have had to use expensive, time-consuming, labour-intensive, and even risky or unpleasant interventions to obtain such a good picture of our physiological state. Now we can wear a device on our wrists, and have the results displayed on our smartphones. Our heart rate variability is a biomarker for many of the diseases caused by stress and lifestyle, which account for at least 70% of disease in the population.

Heart rate variability may also be a key to understanding the many conditions and disorders that we healthcare practitioners refer to resignedly as MUPS (medically unexplained physical symptoms). Our resignation is not only due to the fact that these are so numerous, and that we understand so little about them, but that we have so little to offer in the way of effective treatment.

YOUR HEART RATE VARIABILITY IS UNIQUE

Heart rate variability is unique to each individual person. This means that two people who have the same state of health objectively speaking can have different HRV numbers (different heart rate variability). About 30% of the differences in heart rate variability are genetically determined. The rest are related to one's lifestyle and you can have some influence over this. It is worth noting that people who have endured a traumatic and difficult childhood and adolescence have a lower heart rate variability and a higher stress level and are especially vulnerable to suffering stress disorders and diseases in general. This is why it is important not to compare the numbers you get with those of others. Instead, you should only relate to your own HRV numbers and do it over a period of time. It is also important to know that in general the heart rate variability of women is a little higher than that of men and that heart rate variability decreases with age. As we get older, more activation of the sympathetic nervous system is required for us to maintain the body's functions and capacity for recovery. Heart rate variability can also vary with the seasons and be lower, or worse, in the winter.

It is very important that you understand what heart rate variability is before reading further. Go ahead and look up 'Heart Rate Variability' on YouTube and look through some of the videos you find. If you set aside half an hour to understand what HRV is, you will know more about it than 95% of the Norwegian medical profession.

Lise (28)

I have understood why my partner and I need very different amounts of sleep (and why we have very different energy levels when we both get an equal amount of it). He gets 100 in the Body Battery almost every night while I have to intentionally make sleep a priority if I want to get to the same. He starts charging the moment he sits down and relaxes, even when he drinks beer or wine or after drinking, too. He can drink three or four units of alcohol and still wake up in the morning with a reading of 100. If I want to increase the Body Battery while I am awake, I have to lie completely still, not eat for five hours prior to it, and avoid getting stressed. But even then, we're only talking about going up by 2-3%. If I drink alcohol after midnight, I can just forget about getting over 50 during the night even if I've only had one unit.

The body budget

Do you remember that I mentioned the body budget? We have what you could say is a body budget that contains a certain amount of physiological resources that can be used for physical or mental tasks. Heart rate variability shows us how we deplete or refill our body budget at any one time. When the heart rate variability is high, i.e. during the parasympathetic resting mode, the budget is being replenished and when the heart rate variability is low, i.e. during sympathetic mobilisation, it is being depleted. We draw energy from the same budget no matter what it is – it could be a stressful deadline, a difficult conversation or a rich meal out – that taps us of energy.

The human body is a complex, gigantic organism. It contains an incomprehensible 27 trillion cells, all of which have to be nourished with oxygen and essential nutrients and molecules. The cells send neurotransmitters to each other in an advanced collaborative effort. Immune cells go on patrol and discover problems. Nerve signals hit their mark precisely so that the right muscle cell can be stimulated. Gland cells produce hormones that affect the entire body. The bone marrow produces blood and immune cells. The liver and the kidneys create, transform, detoxify, and excrete substances according to the needs of the body. The skin and mucous membranes protect the insides of our bodies. All these cells are continuously engaged in activities at a hectic pace. Each individual cell contains within itself a small universe of tiny, hard-working molecules and proteins that work around the clock so that we can live. Every inch of our body has an important job to do! And on top of everything – literally – we are equipped with a brain, the universe's most advanced instrument, in which there are 100 billion cells, each one with around 5,000 synapses!

Our entire bodies are, in fact, a temporary composition of primaeval stardust that in this very moment in time forms who we are. The heaviest elements in our molecules originate from neutron stars and supernovas that are billions of years old. Before they became a part of us through the food we eat, they have circulated through the animals, plants, and nature around us, and we are constantly emitting these substances which are then gathered together to be incorporated again into the world around us. We are all a part of a continuous cycle of the decomposition and construction of living material.

As you can probably deduct from the preceding paragraph, everything is connected to everything else, and even though we may look reliable, calm, and solid on the outside, everything is operating at full speed ahead within our inner machinery, which even medical science struggles to comprehend in its entirety. The body budget – about which you will hear quite a lot further on in this book – may therefore remind you less of your manageable, personal financial budget, and more of our infinitely complex global economy.

The impact of both physical and mental stress will appear in your body budget. After engaging in a strenuous mental task, we temporarily become physically weaker. The budget in the body is a shared one, drawn upon from a number of sources, just like it is in many people's own personal budget in which concert tickets, the groceries, car loan payments, a gift for one's spouse, and financial investments are all taken from the same account. And the same is true when it comes to income. Sleep, rest, meditation, and time spent doing constructive activities increase our energies in the same way that depositing our salary or lottery winnings and the savings made by changing to a cheaper telephone service increase the balance in our bank accounts. Up until recently it was hard to know whether your budget was in debit or credit. Now, just like you can see your bank statement on an app on your smartphone, you can have your body budget given to you on heart rate monitors made by Garmin, Oura, WHOOP, and a number of other manufacturers. Their apps can provide you with a picture of the state of your inner energy balance. The currency in your bank is money; the currency of your body budget is your heart rate variability.

The body budget

Lena (59)
I decided to take a break since we were going to travel abroad for a week to go to a wedding. I knew that during that time there would be a lot of alcohol there and we would get little sleep. Taking a break was good, but afterwards I was really motivated to put my watch back on.

HRV monitors and other physiological sensors

Why do we need to use monitors? We need them because our bodies speak softly, and we are poor listeners. If we were able to listen to and interpret the stress within our bodies, then we would have far fewer problems when it comes to balancing our stress and lifestyle-related diseases than we do today. Most of the people who need to pick up the pace in their lives, as well as those who should slow things down, would both have done it by now. Even when our bodies scream out in pain or discomfort, there are many of us who do not listen or pay attention to it. And even when our bodies struggle with just light exertions, there are many of us who fail to take action to improve our strength and fitness.

For millions of years, a natural stress balance was built into the living conditions of our ancestors. It was vital for them to direct their senses and attention out towards the world around them. They hunted and fought when it was necessary to do so, and they rested when they could. They did not really need to have a highly developed sensitivity that enabled them to assess their inner physiological state beyond what was needed to survive (such as dealing with hunger, fatigue, and pain). On the contrary, being more attuned to such things could have ended up disturbing their ability to direct their attention towards external sensory impressions, which was more important for ensuring their survival.

Within us we have a physiological production factory, as well as a transport system that operates on high gear around the clock regardless of whether we notice it or not. Energy is ingested, digested, and consumed without us even so much as registering it. Billions of blood cells are created and destroyed every day. The cacophony of noise from the body's internal drivetrain has to be muted so that we are able to focus our alertness outwards. A submarine does something similar when it has to reduce the noise it makes in order to detect sounds emitted by its enemies. The bustling work of the body continues on easily under the radar. And that is all well and good because if we did notice it then it would be like being in the engine room of the *Titanic* without wearing ear protection.

Reducing the degree of inwardly directed attention was probably advantageous for survival in a far distant time. However, in the times we live in, this does not serve to increase our well-being or ensure our survival. We literally need a support system. By using sensors that measure our heart rate variability, we can compensate for our inadequate ability to sense what is going on inside our bodies. According to psychiatrist Gabor Maté, physiological stress responses are in fact a better measuring stick for gauging what we actually experience than our own conscious and observed behaviours are.

The monitors literally put the control over your health into your own hands. Monitors offer you a better overview of your stress balance than your doctor has access to, even with all the tools at their disposal. This is because for the most part your doctor only has access to measurement results that emerge when an illness has already developed. With a heart rate monitor you can monitor and regulate your health in advance of illness, thereby greatly reducing the likelihood of you being affected by a lifestyle disease. As the healthcare system also becomes aware of the value of these results, then you can report them to your doctor who will more easily be able to assess your state of health. But be prepared: initially your doctor may become annoyed and look down his nose at them.

Heart rate monitors have been in use for many years but for the most part they have been utilised to monitor the efforts athletes make during training as well as their fitness curve. Athletes are entirely dependent on achieving the best possible balance between training and recovery to reach their maximal physiological capabilities. Another important group of people who has put monitors to use is the American military. The soldiers' physical constitution and ability to maintain calm in the midst of extreme, chaotic conditions can be absolutely essential for their survival in war situations. Psychiatrists in the United States and other countries have found that measuring heart rate variability can also help patients who suffer from mental health issues. Therapy can be more effective when a patient's heart rate variability is good, and patients can also detect a worsening of their condition at an early stage and seek help.

The first time I heard about HRV, as recently as 2019, was when I came across it in a book about the treatment of psychological trauma by Bessel van der Kolk entitled *The Body Keeps the Score*. The knowledge that comes out of research environments such as this one now benefits us all.

You can, of course, implement some of the lifestyle-related measures I suggest and not measure the results of doing so at all. However, if you really want to get something out of this book, you should get yourself the tool that allows you access to the main attraction presented here – a guided expedition into your own nervous system.

I have used the last three years to test heart rate monitors and I would like to recommend a few of them here, each one with their own pros and cons. None of the monitors are perfect and you cannot use them to gain control over your nervous system with the same precision that you might find your way through traffic on the road using a GPS, but they are far better than what we have had available to us until now, which was in fact nothing at all.

All the monitors use your heart rate variability to calculate your stress level. Development in this area has been rapid. And even though these measurement systems will doubtless be further developed, using heart rate variability as the measuring stick for assessing one's stress level will remain.

The monitors each have a corresponding app for your smartphone. The apps provide you an overview of the body's state in the moment. They can also compare your progress over a period of days, weeks, months, or years. However, it is one thing to measure your HRV. Just as important as doing that is to place the data into a system that makes it easy for you to follow the results of your changes in lifestyle. Numerous monitors exist on the market which use your pulse and rate of breathing to show your stress level and assess your sleep phases, and which can be used in the implementation of the measures that I am proposing to you. Technology is advancing at such a speed that in a few years there may well be other contenders in the race to improve the balance of your stress and your health other than the ones I mention in the following pages.

> **Heddy Anne (63)**
>
> I work as a coach/psychotherapist and for 20 years have always felt that I love my job. But watching myself go right into resting mode during a session with a client is utterly fantastic! Even while I am engaged in very demanding topics of conversations, I find myself down on a parasympathetic level which is equivalent to a good night's sleep! This tells me something about the value of having good, grounded contact with other people and of being totally present with all my senses directed towards the person in front of me. The same thing happens when I am together with my grandchildren. But as soon as I pick up the phone and start scrolling, the stress increases.

AN OVERVIEW OF VARIOUS MONITORS

Garmin smartwatch

The most affordable and easiest-to-use monitor is the Garmin smartwatch (garmin.com). Perhaps you are one of several million people who are already using one? These watches have a function on them that measures your current stress level based on your heart rate variability. In addition, your accumulated stress load is measured through a feature called the *Body Battery*. Garmin's app is manageable and intuitive. At any given time, the Body Battery energy level number will give you an estimate of which physiological resources you have at your disposal throughout the day.

The most affordable models of heart rate monitors are sufficient for most users, but the big advantage of using the more expensive Garmin models is that they can assess the efforts you make during exercise. This is especially useful for those of you who do not work out regularly because you may have a greater need for recovery after exercise than you think.

The watches can also estimate your fitness level and your biological age, which are among the most important factors for having good health in the future. Your biological age refers to an individual's state of health and ageing, which is not necessarily reflected in our chronological age.

A big, practical advantage of Garmin watches is that the functions can be set so that with a touch of a button you can find out your stress level in the present moment. In this way you can, for example, take a short break to catch your breath and then register the effect of doing so immediately, or observe how long it takes you to settle down after a workout, a stressful situation, or eating a larger meal, and then to find out what effect it has on your body budget.

The people in my test group all used Garmin watches and their experiences can be read throughout this book.

I have also tested watches that compete in the same market as the Garmin such as Apple Watch, Polar and Huawei but these ones do not yet feature the same user-friendly and useful imaging of one's stress level and Body Battery. However, several of the watches do show heart rate variability, sleep quality, and stress level and can definitely be used to carry out the measures in this book.

Recommended energy level numbers on the Body Battery

I would recommend that you try to get the energy level of your Body Battery up to at least 80 in the morning and not under 20 in the evening most days of the week (the scale goes from 5 to 100). If your nervous system has been overburdened over a long period of time or due to very tiring life circumstances, then these energy levels may be difficult to achieve. However, it is exactly in situations such as these that you have a lot to gain by reaching the best possible level you can.

If you struggle to get the Body Battery to read 40 in the morning and regularly end up at 5 in the afternoon or evening, I would take this as a warning sign and I recommend that you follow the advice in this book carefully. If the energy levels still do not increase, you should contact a doctor to rule out an illness being responsible for this.

Oura Ring

Another good option is the Oura Ring (ouraring.com). This is somewhat more expensive than the cheapest Garmin watch, but it is especially good at assessing sleep quality and the different phases of sleep. The Oura Ring also shows a recovery score that tells you if you are ready for a challenging day or not. Each morning you can look at your scores in the app connected to it and, based on what they say, make better decisions when you are looking at the day's tasks ahead of you, such as whether you should take several small breaks or allow yourself to go for an extra run. Maybe you should replace a beer on Friday after work with a non-alcoholic drink and perhaps you could go to bed a little earlier at night.

The Oura Ring will also measure your level of activity and, if you have been sitting still for too long, will suggest that you get up and move around. One minute of running or walking in place would be sufficient. This is an excellent alternative for someone who is not interested in following their stress levels during the day. A big plus with this device is that it is possible to connect it to headphones or ear buds and choose from a big selection of ambient sounds, breathing exercises, and guided meditations. You will also get a figure for the change in heart rate variability during the resting period. In addition, you can have your average heart rate variability recorded during the night.

The ring will give you a good picture of your physiological capacity each morning, and it has a rudimentary daytime stress monitor, but it is not easy to make out what has affected it. In other words, the Oura Ring shows you the balance but not the movement within the accounts. It is quite suitable if you already have a watch that you do not want to replace or if you do not like wearing a watch during the night. It is also ideal if you are afraid that you would get too caught up in keeping up with your data during the day.

Recommended scores for the Oura Ring

You should have a score of 80 for both readiness and for your sleep score most of the days of the week. If you regularly have a score of about 60 for both, then I would consider this to be a warning sign and I would recommend that you follow the advice in this book closely. If the scores do not increase, then you should contact a doctor.

WHOOP bands

The WHOOP band is a fitness and health wearable that attaches around the wrist (whoop.com). In fact, with WHOOP's special undergarments and sportswear you can carry the monitor without it being visible. With WHOOP you pay an annual membership fee so that over time it will cost you more than if you only had a one-time expenditure for a watch or a ring. However, through the membership, WHOOP provides better inter-activity with its users and the information that you enter into it is gathered together and stored. WHOOP assesses how changes in your lifestyle affect your health through weekly and monthly reports.

What WHOOP is especially good at is comparing the scores of your morning recovery with your stress levels during the day in order to be able to recommend how much you should exercise and exert yourself. WHOOP is also good at evaluating your sleep and will indicate your exact sleep requirements calculated relative to your current activity level. The WHOOP app also has a monitor of your stress level for the last 12 hours measured on a scale of 0 to 3. For those of you who have another watch you want to keep using, the WHOOP band can offer you a good alternative to the Oura Ring.

And even if you choose another monitor, you can still enjoy the accumulated knowledge both on WHOOP's website and through what is featured in their podcast series.

Recommended scores for WHOOP

Your recovery score should be in the green zone most days of the week. If you are often in the red zone, then I would consider this to be a red flag and recommend that you follow the advice you find in this book carefully. If your score does not improve, then you should contact a doctor.

Fitbit smartwatches and trackers

The Fitbit is another popular health and activity tracker. While the Fitbit does not show your reserves of energy with quite the same easy visual clarity as the Garmin's Body Battery, the Fitbit PurePulse technology was one of the first wearable heart rate tracking devices, and results for heart rate variability can be found on the Health Metrics dashboard of the Fitbit app. A subscription to Fitbit Premium will give you a 'Daily Readiness Score', which compares your recent activity, sleep, and HRV levels against your personal baseline to assess whether you should prioritise exercise (on high score days, in the 50-70 zone) or recovery (on low-score days, 30 and below).

Smartphone

It is possible to use a mobile phone to take short readings by having the camera phone and the torch function work together to get your heart rate variability. Go to the App Store (iPhone) or Google Play (Android) and search: Heart rate variability camera. A variety of options will appear. HRV4Training (hrv4training.com) is a good one, but I have not tried all the alternatives. Using your phone, you can then take a current snapshot of the state of your nervous system and assess it several times during the day. The downside of using it, of course, is that you cannot track data during the night while you sleep. However, this is a way for you to go through the different stages in the book and use your mobile phone as a measuring device and it will not cost you anything.

YOUR PHYSIOLOGICAL DASHBOARD

Wait, will it be stressful keeping track of my stress?

Many people will certainly wonder if you might go completely crazy by having your eyes glued to these monitors. I don't think so. Most of us are already used to following the latest news online, receiving updates about everything from dramatic international incidents to the love lives of celebrities. What happens in these events is something over which we have no say whatsoever. The reports from inside our bodies, on the other hand, are things that we can in fact influence.

At first it is a little like learning to drive a car. You have to concentrate on looking regularly into the rear-view mirror, checking the road signs, and remembering which driver has the right of way – you or the Volvo that sped up quickly on the right. But by the time you are relatively experienced, and many hundreds of kilometres have disappeared behind you, driving becomes pretty close to being automatic. And then you can listen to a podcast or indulge in a train of complex thoughts and before you know it you have driven a hundred kilometres without noticing it. I think you will experience keeping track of your heart rate variability in the same way. After a while, having an overview of the condition of your body will become as commonplace to you as knowing approximately how much money you have in your bank account, roughly how much the items you usually buy in the shops cost, or how you find your way to an unknown place using a GPS.

But you might be wondering if you will manage to keep track of the scores and numbers. Well, here's a test for you. Are you able to follow what's happening on the dashboard even though you are driving 80 km/h? At that speed, are you able to glance casually at the speedometer or the GPS or check to see if you have enough fuel left to get to where you are going? If you have answered yes, then you can also do this.

Via the car's dashboard we are able to adapt our speed to our surroundings. It would be great to be able to drive at 150 km/h when we want to go somewhere, but it would also be highly risky for ourselves and others. If we drive an equivalent of 150 km/h in physiological speed, it is also risky not only for ourselves but also for those around us. In fact, many states of stress are due to the strain of constantly relating to people who themselves suffer from being out of balance. A frustrated, stressed, and mentally exhausted family member is often the cause of other family members experiencing stress. It might be tempting to try to change the person in question. This rarely helps. And being surrounded by factors causing stress beyond one's control makes it extra vital to focus on the areas that one can in fact have some influence over.

In the same way that we do not have to be perfect drivers to travel safely in public without hurting ourselves and others, but can be just proficient enough, we want to become good drivers of our nervous system. You do not have to chase after the perfect balance. Not only because it is impossible – no one really knows where the balance point lies – but because being good enough will do in this case. Feel free to think of using a monitor as a method for staying on the road – even if you drift a little to the side from time to time, it will prevent you from veering outside the white lines and into the ditch.

What is most essential in this context is to weed out behaviours that are harmful to our health. Just as a pedestrian feels safest when drivers follow the rules of the road, it feels comforting to be with others who have their nervous systems and body budgets in order.

Melina (41)

Wear the monitor for a fair amount of time to get familiar with how different things affect you. Use this as a way to discover yourself or as a way to learn how to be your own guide rather than trying to reach the highest possible score. Don't get stressed out thinking that you have to follow all of the scores and data every single day. Go at your own pace!

Eventually you won't need to track all the data. You will learn when it is the right time to check your status. Make small changes to check whether they are having an effect on your sleep quality, stress level, etc.

From low energy and stress to a surplus of energy and peace of mind

Although having a good balance in your physiology will reduce your risk of contracting a number of diseases, the aim of this book is equally to gain a mental and physical surplus of energy for your everyday life in the here and now. This improves your ability to take on challenges and take care of and make use of the opportunities before you. In a way, a good physiology is like fresh fruit: the surplus energy we get from getting quality sleep can 'go off' during the course of a couple of days, and muscular strength can wither away in just a few weeks. If we work against our physiology, then we are doomed to fail.

Being in balance and having a surplus of energy provide you with strength and the willpower to live your life the way you choose. When you feel low it is difficult to find the energy needed to make good decisions. This in turn increases the deficit you are experiencing. A downward spiral thus begins. And one of the first things to fall by the wayside when we are stuck in a deficit energy mode is our willpower. The state of our willpower is closely connected to our heart rate variability. Studies have shown that those people who have the best heart rate variability resist temptation with greater ease. Research conducted to test alcoholics' responses has proven this. HRV scores can in fact predict which of the sober alcoholics will be the first to give in to the temptation of having a drink. The best state to be in to gain access to your willpower is when your heart rate settles down and your heart rate variability increases. That's when we feel balanced and focused, and we can then make well-considered choices. People with a higher heart rate variability are better at delaying gratification, coping with stress, ignoring distractions, and exercising self-control.

Remember to be patient with yourself. Being impatient is often the worst character flaw of those who tend to overwork themselves. These people want to recover and get healthy yesterday, and the slow improvement to their health frustrates them to no end. No one, however, is capable of forcing a state of recovery and rest to occur in the same way that we can mobilise our resources to make a vigorous effort. All we can do is facilitate favourable conditions for recovery to take place. The good news is that becoming patient is something we can work on, and while you wait for your health to improve, you can exercise your patience muscles. Feel free to practise this in your everyday life. Look forward to standing in the queue at the shop, in traffic, on the telephone or, best of all, my favourite, at the airport.

Think of learning to master your physiology as being like learning to play the violin. If you become frustrated by your slow progress, consider this: how long would it take to be good enough to play Bach and Beethoven in front of a big audience? And when you realise that your body is a far more complex instrument than a violin, then you can pat yourself on the back for every little step you make in the way of progress. I myself continue to learn something new every single day, and I am more than three years in to following my nervous system closely. Obviously, I wish for both you and everyone else the quickest possible path to recovery and improved health, but it is actually far more important how improved your state of health will be six months from now, and for the rest of your life.

The problem is that we are all used to getting quick results. We order things online and are able to get them delivered to our door the next day. We wonder about something, and Google provides an answer pretty much the moment the thought arises. In films, life's problems are solved within a couple of hours. However, in the real world even small changes can take a long time. The actual decision to make a change, though, often comes suddenly – and when you have decided to make a change, a lot has already been accomplished. So even though the distance from where you are to where you want to go seems far, now you are on the path to recovery you can tell yourself encouragingly that you are exactly where you are supposed to be!

Suggested reading

The Power of Patience: How This Old-Fashioned Virtue Can Improve Your Life by M.J. Ryan

The Willpower Instinct: How Self-Control Works, Why It Matters, and What You Can Do to Get More of It by Kelly McGonigal

---

Siri (44)

My heart rate monitor is worth its weight in gold. Stress and lack of sleep have burnt me out and when I caught Covid in January 2021, my entire system crashed and then worsened with Omicron a year later. I am still struggling with the side effects.

The heart rate monitor with the Body Battery gives me a number that tells me how much energy I have at my disposal during the day. It correlates rather well with how I actually feel. During the first period that I used it, the Body Battery energy level number was often around 5 or 6 already quite early in the evening. I have noticed that I have to be aware when the number is under 20 because I then become more tired, irritable, less patient, and I have a shorter fuse. I ought to just unwind, do peaceful activities, such as practising mindfulness or reading a book. I have got much better at this after clearly seeing the consequences of what I do.

I am quite familiar with sleep advice and sleep hygiene, but people think that they already know all about it. With a watch you can see the effect of it directly, and then it is much easier to make a change. I quickly understood that the quality of my sleep was deteriorating because I was too active. My heart rate monitor, and what I have read and learnt about it, have made it so that I am finally able to move in the right direction after many years of being frustrated and suffering from chronic stress, which has a lot to do with my family life. There are some factors that I am not completely in control of, but the watch helps me to feel better in several areas. In general, I push myself too hard and I am not very good at relaxing, recovering, or taking breaks. And to a greater degree I have realised that I should take into

From low energy and stress to a surplus of energy

account that eating late meals, exercising, and drinking alcohol worsen my sleep.

    Lately I have managed to get the Body Battery above 20 when I go to bed. Whereas I could have woken up in the morning with the Body Battery down to around 40 to 50 before, now it is often at 70 to 80. I have a way to go, but the numbers are positive, and I think that the important changes I am making in my lifestyle will help me get into better shape.

THE
PRACTICE

Thank you for your patience in getting through the theory presented here! Now that you have hopefully received some answers to things you may have been wondering about, you are finally ready to embark on this expedition. And if you don't feel quite ready, that's OK, because that is not vital. Based on my experience I would say that it pays to start before you are ready, otherwise you may never begin, and I say this from hard-won wisdom. The most important thing is to just get going; you can make adjustments along the way. So, grab your Oura Ring, Garmin watch, WHOOP band, Fitbit, or download a HRV app and get out your mobile phone. The first step is the most important one.

I wish you welcome as a fellow participant on this expedition! Get your well-being, willpower, and mental and physical health ready for a reboot. Fasten your seatbelt, release the handbrake, and hold onto your hat!

Discover your starting point

It pays to begin with a reality orientation. I suggest that you make an assessment of where you are right now. As soon as you know where you are, then it becomes easier to estimate the distance to your goal. This is like deciding which road you are going to take on a map app: the distance to be covered only becomes known to you after you have entered the starting point and the journey's end. And we all have different starting points and goals. You do not have to fill in the forms on the following pages to start the recovery process, but doing so might turn out to be very helpful for you.

If you are exhausted, depressed, or have pain or other bodily ailments, then I would advise you to visit your GP first in order to rule out any of these being caused by a medical condition that should be treated. Below I have listed all the tests everyone should take. Your doctor may add others.

RECOMMENDED MEDICAL TESTS

- **Blood pressure:** Feel free to buy a home blood pressure monitor. Many people's blood pressure is higher when they are at their doctor's practice than it is in their usual, everyday lives, and often a home monitor shows a lower level. If you take blood pressure medication, you may, judging by your findings when testing at home, need less than the dosage indicated via the doctor's measurements. Many people are afraid that using a home monitor will make them stressed, but my experience is just the opposite. The more control my patients feel that they have over their situation, the more at ease they become.

- **Blood tests:**
  (Be aware that you can have symptoms of deficiency even if your values of vitamin B12, vitamin D, folic acid and ferritin are within normal ranges. The optimal level for your health can be quite a lot higher than the lower end of the normal range. Consult your doctor for advice.)
  Vitamin B12. The value should be over 400. A value under this can indicate a deficiency.
  Folic acid
  Metabolism: Ft 4 and TSH
  Vitamin D. The value should be over 80. A value under this can indicate a deficiency.
  Iron. The ferritin level should be over 50. A level under this can indicate a deficiency.
  Sedimentation rate (ESR)
  Fasting blood sugar (glucose) – preferably under 6mmol/L
  Long-term blood sugar (HbA1c) – preferably under 42

Hanne (32)
My friend has a chronic vitamin B12 deficiency, and she needs injections to keep the level of it up. And she discovered an obvious connection between the Body Battery before and after taking B12 supplements. Previously, she waited far too long before taking a supplement, but now she can look at the Body Battery when it is time for a new injection.

Health form
This short survey will show you the present state of your health. Go ahead and take this survey again after you have finished this book. At that time, use a different coloured pen so you can easily see the changes that have taken place.

PHYSICAL AND MENTAL STATES

Scale: How often do feel that you have . . .

0 = never, 1 = almost never, 2 = sometimes, 3 = quite often, 4 = very often.
Circle the number that best matches your state.

Positive mental states

Good willpower:	0	1	2	3	4
Peace of mind:	0	1	2	3	4
Patience:	0	1	2	3	4
Meaningful days:	0	1	2	3	4
Surplus energy:	0	1	2	3	4
Control over your everyday life:	0	1	2	3	4
Feeling a zest for life:	0	1	2	3	4
Positive stress/a good state of being active and engaged:	0	1	2	3	4
Enthusiasm:	0	1	2	3	4
Totals:					

Negative mental states

Irritation:	0	1	2	3	4
Anger:	0	1	2	3	4
Loneliness:	0	1	2	3	4
Sadness:	0	1	2	3	4
Negative stress:	0	1	2	3	4
Worrying:	0	1	2	3	4
Anxiety:	0	1	2	3	4
Totals:					

Physical symptoms

Headaches:	0	1	2	3	4
Physical pain:	0	1	2	3	4
Digestive disorders:	0	1	2	3	4
Rash:	0	1	2	3	4
Fatigue:	0	1	2	3	4
Symptoms of chronic disease:	0	1	2	3	4
Dizziness:	0	1	2	3	4
Totals:					

PHYSICAL CAPACITY

Scale: 0 = weak/poor, 1 = fairly weak/poor, 2 = OK, 3 = fairly strong/good, 4 = very strong/good.
Circle the number that best matches your condition.

Upper body muscular strength:	0	1	2	3	4
Lower body muscular strength:	0	1	2	3	4
Condition:	0	1	2	3	4
Balance:	0	1	2	3	4
Agility:	0	1	2	3	4
Flexibility:	0	1	2	3	4
Totals:					

LIFESTYLE FACTORS

Scale: 0 = very dissatisfied, 1 = dissatisfied, 2 = somewhat satisfied, 3 = quite satisfied, 4 = very satisfied.
Circle the number that best matches your state.

Sleep quality:	0	1	2	3	4
Stress level:	0	1	2	3	4
The ability to rest:	0	1	2	3	4
Activity/exercise level:	0	1	2	3	4
Diet:	0	1	2	3	4
Alcohol consumption:	0	1	2	3	4
Totals:					

How to change bad habits

In the following chapters you are going to learn about changing habits, preferably those stemming from life-long patterns that seem unconquerable and inbuilt. I myself thought, as I was told, that habits are nearly impossible to change and that I just had to accept the bad ones. I thought that the weight accumulated around my waist was an inevitable part of growing older and that my personality was permanently fixed. However, during the last five or six years I have been able to change my lifestyle entirely, with great impact on my mental and physical well-being. I will tell you more about this transformation further on in this book. If I can make changes, then so can you. Although it did not happen in the blink of an eye, these changes were still easier to pull off than you might think. The first commandment to follow is to stop listening to those who say it is difficult. At least for me, enacting change was much easier to do after I had stopped believing it was difficult.

The most important consequence of developing a good habit is that it can replace willpower. Using our willpower drains us of energy and a little is depleted with every single choice we make. The more that your day's intelligent responses to situations can come from the category of 'habits', the more willpower you can save and reallocate for other challenges. Here lies a paradox: willpower is required to change habits which in their turn reduce the need for willpower. But as soon as you have entered a positive flow, each step going in the right direction will be strengthened and it will give you increased energy. Forming one good habit can make it easier to rid yourself of other bad habits.

You do not necessarily need to completely alter your habits – often adjusting them suffices. Can you sleep a little better, eat a little more healthily, be stressed out a little less, exercise a little more, drink a little less alcohol, and rest a little more? If you remove a few temptations from your surroundings, then maybe you can avoid using less energy to resist them? Small changes often have the biggest effect, and the combined value of these minor adjustments are perhaps all that is needed to make a difference!

Anita (58)
Be patient and do one thing at a time. It takes time to become familiar with old patterns that are really ingrained. This is not a quick fix; it is a change in lifestyle.

12 tips for making a successful change in lifestyle

To gain control over our inner fossil, we need assistance from our intellect, our thinking frontal lobe, to get traction. What follows are the most important coping techniques you need to make lasting lifestyle changes.

1. **Accept things as they are.** Being frustrated due to having an injustice inflicted on you steals energy from you and hinders you from moving on. When you accept the situation as it is, you liberate energy that can be used for recovering or healing.
2. **Be grateful.** Possessing a general gratefulness for what you have increases your chances of receiving more to be grateful for.
3. **Set goals for yourself** that are concrete, measurable, achievable, and that preferably have a deadline.
4. **Make the most out of the difficulties you face** and use them to learn and grow.
5. **Take responsibility.** Take 100% responsibility for whatever happens to you. That includes absolutely everything. That is how

you can wrestle control over your own life from the circumstances
you find yourself in, and all the excuses you have had will cease to
be valid.

6. **Learn from mistakes.** Value the mistakes that are able to bring
   you closer to your goal (as long as you learn from them). In order
   to do more of the right things, you have to dare to make more
   mistakes.

7. **Seize the moment.** Be present in the here and now with your
   whole being. Take hold of opportunities when you see them.

8. **Stop chasing perfection.** Being good enough is more than
   sufficient. Facing situations with this attitude, you will take more
   chances, and you will benefit from it.

9. **Prepare for luck to strike.** Luck happens when preparation meets
   opportunity. Bad luck strikes those who are inattentive or unpre-
   pared, who ignore or only spot opportunities after they have
   passed them by.

10. **Find meaning in what you do.** What is the most meaningful thing
    you can spend your life doing?

11. **Compose your life.** What would you like to have more of in your
    life? What can you cast aside? Use your time and energy on what
    nourishes you, instead of what wears you down.

12. **Follow your dreams.** Life is too short to waste shuffling through
    days that are dull and uneventful. Make your everyday life a party
    or head out on an adventure – and if possible, take someone
    with you!

The approaches above can be used to implement lifestyle changes as well
as for other changes required of us by the challenges life sends our way.
The peace of mind, the resilience, and the coping skills you will have
acquired can take you a long way.

As you know I am a keen photographer, and over the years, having
taught workshops all over the world, I have learnt that the best photographers know two methods for improving: taking tiger leaps and mouse
steps. Those people who do not succeed only know about the former.

Sure, sometimes you have to take a tiger leap and make a big effort or dare to do something you fear, but the most important thing we can do is to take tiny steps forward. These small, seemingly insignificant mouse steps that head in the right direction, taken together, constitute the foundation for success.

The tiny, daily, good choices that we make are easy to take and yet easy to drop altogether. When looked at individually they are almost invisible, both to ourselves and to others. But over time they can snowball into something known as the compound effect. Over time the small, comfortable choices will weaken you and make you feel unpleasant, while the small, uncomfortable choices you make will trigger your resilience and you will create a different kind of comfort in the long run.

Being kind or compassionate towards oneself has proven to be more important than self-confidence for a person's quality of life. If you are the type of person who beats yourself up as soon as you make a mistake, then you decrease your chances for succeeding at what you do and of thriving. Therefore, it is important to be someone you can say supportive things to. Be your own best friend and be the one who can help you the most! You are free of charge, always nearby, and motivated to make the effort. Many of my patients struggle dealing with a lousy inner assistant. The voice inside tells them that they aren't worth anything, they will never make it, things will never go well, they are not good enough to succeed, they do not deserve to get better, and they might as well give up.

If you recognise yourself as being at the mercy of these thought patterns, it is a signal that you need a partner with you during this recovery process. Thoughts of this nature are delusional and can be corrected, but in the meantime you need an honest soul by your side who wants you to get better and dares to give you some resistance, someone with empathy and who is responsible.

Recommended reading

The Power of Habit: Why We Do What We Do and How to Change by Charles Duhigg

Atomic Habits: An Easy & Proven Way to Build Good Habits & Break Bad Ones by James Clear

Heddy Anne (63)
Now I have learnt more about how I can take care of my health a little better. I have always thought that I was responsible for myself, but now it is perhaps a little easier to take this responsibility on.

A trick for getting started

If you, as soon as the topic of making a change in your life comes up, easily resort to platitudes such as 'old habits are hard to break', 'it is easier said than done', and 'that is easy for you to say', then I have a suggestion for you. Write these clichés down, each one on their own separate piece of paper. Crumple all of them together and throw them in the rubbish bin. Ingrained fallacies such as these can sabotage your entire process for making changes. Replace them with positive statements such as 'practice makes perfect', 'one step at a time', or 'seek and ye shall find'. Remember that what you say to yourself tends to happen.

A little about the stages of this expedition

For most people, including myself, it comes as a great shock suddenly to gain insight into the state of our nervous systems. Therefore, it may be a good idea for us to proceed quite calmly. During the first two weeks of this expedition, live exactly as you have up until now. Follow the results without getting too hung up on them. Try to accept that this is a reflection of how your nervous system works at the moment. Make a note of interesting observations or data that surprise you, and jot down findings you would like to change or keep, but during this time, you do not need to change anything at all.

It would be helpful to keep a diary or, even better, a designated health journal. Then you can compare your sleep quality and your efforts through the day with the numbers you get from your device. While going over the theory and mapping out your situation, you may find one or more areas where you are struggling in particular. Maybe you should begin with making some changes there? Or would you prefer to focus on an area that would present a less laborious task so that you have a greater chance to succeed? Some people like to acclimatise themselves gradually and others want to jump in at the deep end right away. Approach this the way that suits you the best!

The chapters in this book have been placed in an order based on, judging from my experience as a doctor, what is most important to most people. I reckon that two weeks spent working on each stage would be a good use of your time. However, feel free to go through the chapters in the sequence and at the pace you feel best for you. You can also keep going to the next stage even if you have not quite completed the goal of the previous one because, such are the connections between the physiology and the autonomic nervous system, the solution to an issue you have encountered in a previous stage may in fact be found in the next.

> **Emilie (31)**
> The Body Battery numbers have given me a completely new understanding of how everything is connected! Day and night influence each other and many of the small choices that I make during the day have a great effect. This knowledge is the basis for the power to make changes!

13 factors that affect one's body budget

The five big stages:

1. Sleep
2. Stress
3. Movement and exercise
4. Active rest
5. Meals and diet
6. The hippo: alcohol

In addition, there are some stages that will apply only to some of you reading this book:

7. Illness and disease
8. Weight control
9. Nicotine

And finally, here are some predetermined factors:

10. Age
11. Seasonal variation

12. Gender
13. Menstruation

I have divided each stage into four parts:

1. The science
2. From the doctor's practice
3. My exploration
4. Your exploration

The science: In this section I will extract the essence from hundreds of relevant books I have read as well as hundreds of podcasts and videos that contain the most current knowledge on a topic. Fortunately, there is now a short distance between scientific discoveries and their effective dissemination. When I studied medicine in the 1990s, we heard hardly a single word about sleep, fasting, exercise, obesity, intestinal flora, inactivity, stress or relaxation techniques. Dietary advice had major shortcomings and the concept of preventative medicine was all but non-existent. The study of lifestyle diseases had not yet been included in the curriculum. However, during the last 20 years the quantity of knowledge about these subjects has exploded. There are more researchers, the instruments are better, and technology has made it easier to collect and analyse large amounts of data and then publicise the findings through YouTube channels and podcasts. General knowledge about the topics in this book is so extensive that in order to write this book I had to read five times as much as I did in all the six years of my medical studies. Obviously, I want to make this knowledge as concise and easy for you to read as possible. Therefore, I have summarised concepts when I could, but will direct you towards popular science books that can tell you more if you want to read further.

In tandem with reading this book I recommend you make use of your free time to listen to podcasts about topics found here, perhaps when you are driving your car, doing housework, or going for a walk. The two podcasts I recommend that you listen to in particular are *Feel Better, Live More* with Dr Rangan Chatterjee and *The Diary of a CEO*, in which host

Steven Bartlett frequently interviews health professionals. The WHOOP podcast is also well worth a listen. These podcasts are committed to exploring and finding out how a person can take action on their own to improve their health. You will also be able to find many more great podcasts listed in the back of this book.

From the doctor's practice: In this part I will relate the first-hand experiences I have had with my patients at my practice, also known as empirical data. Over the years I have conducted over 100,000 consultations. That does not mean that all the conclusions I have drawn are absolute. Certainly, it could well be that another doctor whose base of experience is as broad as mine would come to different conclusions. Despite this, I will share my clinical experience here.

As a rule, before I sit down with a patient, I start by going over their medical history, often going back several years. Even if the person has this time come in because of a troublesome toe, an attentive doctor would be able to place this problem into a larger context through his or her overview of the patient's total state of health. Often, other members of a patient's family also attend the same doctor's practice, and this may help clarify the patient's situation even more. Parents come in with their child and in time this grown child will return with his or her grandparents. Not infrequently, the practice is full of relatives. In addition, when we often make home visits, we are able to see the environment that the patients live in.

After working for 15 years as a doctor, the feeling of discomfort I mentioned earlier began to creep in. I was learning and experiencing something I had not covered during my studies: most of the diseases that I treated, and the medications I prescribed for them, were rooted in poor lifestyle choices. These choices had become so familiar for my patients that they seemed like the normal thing for them to do in certain circumstances. What many of them had in common was an imbalance in their stress systems, which, as you have now understood, can be measured in their heart rate variability.

My exploration: In this part you will get to hear what I have learnt about my own autonomic nervous system after looking at data daily using several devices for over three years. Through this I am going to show how the state of the nervous system and physiology can be judged in the readings we take. Even though the factors that affect us as people are all the same, we as individuals are unique and we all react differently to the same factors. Therefore, the results I have do not represent a standard or ideal to strive for. On the contrary, I still have the potential for improvement even after making a lot of adjustments.

Most of us have a moment when we wake up to the state of our health. When I was in my 30s and early 40s, I was so occupied with working and making money so I could afford to sail around the world with my family that I completely neglected my health. It was not until my father died unexpectedly at the age of 73 that I began to take a good look at myself in the mirror. What I saw was not exactly uplifting. I was overweight, out of shape, malnourished, and overworked. I smoked, used snus (snuff – very commonly used in Norway), slept too little, and drank too much alcohol. To top it all off, I was a doctor, and I should have known better. I was on a steady course to contract the lifestyle diseases that I knew all too well from the time I had spent with my patients.

I had two alternatives: undergo a gruelling transformation of my health now or pay the price in the form of being ill, taking medication, having a reduction in my quality of life, and having my lifespan shortened. I decided on initiating an immediate reversal of my situation. I managed to do this. I got into better shape and within a couple of years I was able to lose 20 kilos that I did not need. My level of energy increased, and I felt much better about myself. And I am certain that if I had not managed to change my lifestyle, I would have ended up having the same lifestyle diseases that I get paid to treat.

When I began measuring my heart rate variability three years ago, I felt as if I was fumbling around in the dark. I read some data or a curve and tried to connect it to what I was feeling in my body. Now, when I try to follow what is happening in my body, I can predict quite precisely which stress level I'm at and how my heart rate variability curve varies throughout the day. Being able to perceive the nuances between the feeling of stress and having surplus energy took me a long time to do. I have also spent a good deal of time mapping how the various stresses – common stress, work, diet, exercise, disease, or stimulants such as alcohol or nicotine – impact my body, and just as much energy exploring how alleviating and restorative factors such as sleep, rest, meditation, breathing exercises, cold showers, and fasting can compensate for the stresses. I hope that the work I have done here will streamline your own exploration of physiology, the nervous system, and the body budget.

Your exploration: In this part I will offer some advice about how you can work with the stage in question. All of the words written in this book would be rendered meaningless if they didn't lead *you* towards having a better life. I have already experienced the benefit of using the monitors and I have reaped the rewards of doing so. Now you are the one who is centre stage! If you are like most people, you will be able to uncover some hidden thieves of your energy and find new ways to increase your surplus of it. Not least, you will discover the security that exists in having knowledge about the fluctuations in your personal body battery. If you happen to be one of the fortunate ones whose data shows that there is no need for you to make any changes, you can rejoice in the fact that you have made good life choices and that you can pass this book on to someone who needs it more than you do.

I am painfully aware of how difficult it can be to make changes in your life. However, I also know that making changes is much easier to accomplish when the results can be measured. This 'unfortunately' involves taking a reality orientation as to what your actual situation is. Realising the truth of the situation starts by collecting facts. What you can measure can more easily be mastered! But, yes, there is a lot of effort connected to working actively to change your lifestyle. Still, I have witnessed at my practice that *not* doing anything is great deal more arduous. You can see this as a choice between investing regularly in future health benefits with generous returns or abandoning your efforts and putting yourself into a health-related debt that has to be paid off with exorbitant interest over a period of time. Unfortunately, many people end up going bankrupt. I myself try to go by the rule of thumb to invest one hour a day in various initiatives and activities that invigorate me and prolong my life. But you can choose for yourself how great of an effort you want to put into this. Right now, the main point here for you is to get a better overview of your current body budget. It will become easier to allocate your resources when you know how much energy it costs you to put forth an effort or how much energy you can accumulate through resting.

Mastery in partnership

We are at our best when we master something in partnership with others. Through evolution we have been designed to function this way, and this has been proven not least through making changes in exercise and diet and through quitting smoking. Go ahead and enlist a friend or two to join forces with you so that you can learn from each other's experiences as well as have fun together. Maybe you know someone who is adept at something you need help with and maybe you know something that another person would like to master.

The goal is not to end up in a constant state of living perfectly balanced, monotonous days. The aim is to live in such a way that our nervous systems become flexible and can alternate between complete calm and very intense activity. During some days and weeks, we have to give everything we have and push ourselves to the outer limits of our powers. This is not a cause for concern; we just have to make sure we are equally skilled at picking ourselves up and recovering afterwards. If we go through our days either at a uniformly high speed or steadily idling, we lose our flexibility. The most important thing here for us is to gain control over our stress balance and avoid it becoming primarily influenced by someone else's agenda.

The part of the expedition that can be done from the comfort of an armchair is hereby complete. I hope that along the way you have gathered a lot of knowledge and felt your motivation increase because now we are going to hit the road!

Get to know your body better

As you measure your stress level, try to sense what is going on in your body. Is there a connection between the two? Other times you can try to estimate your stress level *before* you read your monitor. Be patient because it takes time to experience the connection between the two.

Hanne (21)

I have ME/CFS and it clearly affects my nervous system. And even though I am bedridden almost constantly, I am in the orange on my Garmin watch nearly all my waking hours. Because of ME, small things have a big impact on my nervous system. If I am standing brushing my teeth, my heart rate is 150, and if I am sitting in a chair talking to someone it can get as high as 130 to 140. If I am lying stretched out on my bed, as a rule I am around 80 to 90. If I want to get down to 70, then I will have had to have a lot of rest, so I was very surprised when one day I sat singing softly while strumming a guitar by the fact that I was down to around 70! If I sit completely still on a chair, I am in the orange, but if I begin to sing or play guitar then I usually go straight to the blue. That's really strange because you would think I would use more energy singing and playing than just sitting quietly. But it seems as if the effects of mindfulness make up for all of the energy I use sitting doing something. Lying on the bed listening to music produces the same effect.

The stages

In Africa they talk about the Big Five: elephants, lions, rhinoceroses, leopards, and water buffaloes. These are the five big game animals that represent the biggest challenge to hunt on foot. The word 'challenge' might also describe the five stages we are about to embark on: good sleep, better stress balance, higher activity levels, effective rest, and proper diet. The greater the challenge the greater the victory will be when we succeed!

STAGE ONE: SLEEP

The world record for staying awake without sleep is 11 days. It is a record that will never be challenged; sleep deprivation is so dangerous that *The Guinness Book of Records* has not allowed any new record attempts since 1989. You can climb 1,000 metres up a vertical rockface without any safety rope or drive a rocket car at 1,000 km/h – but to go without sleep is too risky.

All the body's vital systems, tissues, and organs suffer damage when we get too little sleep. Many of the most common, life-threatening diseases in industrialised countries, including cardiovascular disease, obesity, diabetes, dementia, and cancer, have a known causal relationship with sleep deprivation. The less you sleep, the shorter your life expectancy.

Other negative side effects include loss of motivation, memory loss, and mood swings. With improved sleep patterns you will have more energy – all the more important as you launch on this book's next challenges. Which is why we'll start here!

Ellen (58)

I find sleeping difficult! For someone like me who has struggled with sleep and stress-related illnesses for 25 years, it has been interesting to be able to see what affects me during the night by following along with a heart rate monitor. All my activities during the day – eating, fasting, exercise, meditation, socialising, drinking alcohol and being on a holiday – play their part. It is also fascinating to see how differently the various activities play out in the data from person to person, how an acquaintance of mine without any specific issues can get completely different numbers to someone who is as sensitive as I am.

The science

Every living organism, even an amoeba, has a circadian rhythm. All more complex animals have a sleep-like recovery state. Were sleep not so important, evolution would not have allowed anything so risky to develop; animals are extra vulnerable to attack while in a state of unconsciousness.

There is still much about the function of sleep that we do not understand. But one thing is certain: sleep is extremely important for human function and health.

Two-thirds of all adults in industrialised countries sleep less than the recommended eight hours per night. This is a disaster waiting to happen: poor sleep increases the risk of various diseases, reduces fertility, makes us dangerous behind the wheel and ineffective at work. For an athlete the risk of injury is increased, while the recovery of their muscles and cells is reduced. Lack of sleep is said to have contributed to several major accidents at nuclear facilities, as well as shipping disasters with large oil spills.

The benefits of a good night's sleep are numerous, and include higher energy levels, better concentration and learning capacity, stronger willpower, an increased ability to make healthy food choices, a stronger immune system, more efficient autophagy (the degradation or repair of damaged cells), lower risk of obesity, lower stress levels – and, not least, a reduced risk of Alzheimer's disease, cancer, heart disease, and other conditions whose underlying cause is chronic inflammation.

Sleep is divided into four phases that roll in cycles of approximately 90 minutes. In the first phase, we experience deep sleep (non-REM, where REM stands for *Rapid Eye Movement*). It is in this phase that 95% of the growth hormone is released into the blood to replace and repair our cells. Throughout the rest of the night, we experience cycles of REM sleep, which improve memory and concentration. It is during this phase that our imaginative dreams generally occur. Each period of REM sleep is longer than the last, the longest usually coming just before we get up in the morning. It is this vital phase of sleep that we can miss if we get up too soon. Between these important phases, we experience light sleep and occasional awakenings, often so short we are unaware of them.

During sleep the pressure in the brain is lowered. Our brain cells shrink and the space between them makes room for a recently discovered system by which waste matter from the day's brain work is flushed away. The accumulation of such substances seems to be a significant cause of dementia and several other diseases affecting the brain.

Regular sleep routines are important for sleep efficiency. It appears that the brain falls more easily into a rhythm for deep sleep and REM sleep if we go to bed and get up at roughly the same time each day. We should go to sleep at around 10.00 p.m., because the early part of sleep is particularly effective for restitution. This is probably because the brain is evolutionarily adapted to go to sleep at this time.

Every cell in the body and brain has a built-in circadian clock which ensures that it functions optimally at different times of the day, depending on the task it is assigned. Sleep recovery, for example, works best at night, while the bowels work best during the day.

The opposite of a regular circadian rhythm – shift work – is as dangerous as smoking and is one of the biggest health risks to which we can be exposed. It can in fact reduce life expectancy by up to 15 years. In Denmark shift work is classified as carcinogenic, yet the financial reward given to health workers and other workers for night work does not compensate for these harmful consequences. Sadly, one in five European workers works shifts and is thus in the danger zone.

Sleep advice for shift work

Many important jobs unavoidably involve night work. Working shifts can be very harmful to your health and create inflammation. The British doctor Rangan Chatterjee gives the following advice to everyone who works at night: expose yourself to strong light during the evening or night while you are working. Limit your exposure to light in the morning after you get off work. Use glasses that reduce blue light. In order to raise your cortisone level, which keeps you alert and healthy, it may be smart to work out before your night shift. Eat more proteins and fewer carbohydrates during the night. Try to sleep as soon as you get home. Eat in a 12-hour window such as starting at 7.00 p.m. and not after 7.00 a.m. so that your daytime sleep can be more restorative.

Vibeke (49)
You can easily get hung up on having poor numbers, and feeling like you have failed can negatively impact your psyche. My best tool is to accept the data and make a plan for the next day. A night of poor sleep, that's fine, then I will adjust my tasks accordingly without making a big deal about it. I create a good day using the starting point I have there and then.

Suggested reading
Why We Sleep: The New Science of Sleep and Dreams by Matthew Walker
The Circadian Code: Lose Weight, Supercharge Your Energy and Sleep Well Every Night by Dr Satchin Panda

From the doctor's practice

Insomnia is a regular visitor at doctors' practices. This is evidenced by the number of prescriptions we hand out for sleeping tablets. When I ask my patients about their sleep patterns, the answer is rarely positive, regardless of what illness or condition they might be struggling with. Many describe waking in the night or difficulty falling asleep. Others wake before the cockerel crows and can't get back to sleep. Many start the working day in a state of exhaustion and wake up as tired as they did when they went to bed. In line with the population's weight gain, others are also affected by sleep apnoea – a disorder where the sufferer snores heavily and their breathing stops and starts during the night. This results in a low oxygen count in the blood, disrupted sleep cycles, and excess stress on the heart. With the rising numbers in people living alone, it is increasingly difficult to pick up on snoring or respiratory cessation at night. Reflux is another weight-related problem at night: excess fat around the trachea and visceral fat that exerts pressure on the lungs make it easier for stomach acid to rise into the oesophagus. This often leads to repeated awakenings or other discomforts that reduce the quality of sleep.

People often try very hard to fall asleep and get frustrated when they fail. This is rarely useful. The adrenaline and cortisol released when we get anxious or irritated about our inability to sleep can in fact keep us awake. The more we chase sleep, the further it slips from our grasp. A better approach is to prepare for and *allow* sleep to come. This is easier when the nervous system is in balance and the resting heart rate is calm. That is why it is so important to wind down in the evening before going to bed.

Good sleep at night is created during the day. The day's stresses can impinge on our night. A poor night's sleep demands, in turn, that we mobilise more energy to function the next day. This creates a downward spiral.

Many people live such busy lives, it is only in those moments after going to bed that they are calm enough to let the thoughts they have suppressed all day come to the surface. Concerns about the near and distant future fill the darkness and prevent sleep. Ultimately, it could be a lack of sleep that tips someone into burnout.

> **Lars (53)**
> I rarely wake up with the Body Battery at 100 when I am sleeping indoors, but when I sleep outside in a hammock or in a car with the doors open, it happens quite often. I think it might have something to do with fresh, cool air. The stress levels are somewhat lower when I'm sleeping outdoors.

My exploration

There will be time enough to sleep when I'm dead! That was how I thought until a few years ago. Getting good-quality and abundant sleep was at the bottom of my mile-long to-do list. I had also developed a habit of having a glass of red wine in the evening, with the idea that it would help me sleep better. Alcohol has since proven to be the worst sleep-killer. Continual changes to my working hours, going from day shifts, to evening or night shifts, put my circadian rhythm into disarray.

I once thought that a stressful day would lead to a correspondingly deep sleep at night, that falling asleep in an exhausted heap would result in better sleep than if I'd had a quiet day. My homespun theory was wrong. My data shows that rest, particularly in the final two hours before bed, is vital for effective sleep. The body and the brain take time to calm down before the 'restoration switch' is ready to be turned on. That's why I now try to take it easy in the last couple of hours before bed. I dim the light and avoid eating or exercise – and find myself a book instead. I have come up with three techniques that help me to fall asleep more quickly:

1. Breathe in a calming rhythm: four seconds on inhalation and six seconds on exhalation.
2. Read a suitably dull academic e-book on my iPhone, with white text on a black background. My room is then totally dark, and I can rarely read more than 10 or 20 pages before my eyelids start to droop – and if I still can't sleep, I can at least benefit from my

reading and so curb the vicious cycle of frustration at not getting to sleep. I purposely avoid exciting books that make me curious about what's on the next page, or that describe riveting events in people's lives.

3. If I can't sleep after putting my iPhone down, I count to 100 in my head. If I get to 100 and am still awake, I start again. This prevents thoughts going round in my head. To ensure I get the last important cycles of REM sleep, I try to avoid getting up too early in the morning: 8.30 a.m. or later is ideal.

Before I started using heart rate monitors, I had no way of knowing the actual quality of my sleep, let alone what affected it. One of the first things heart rate monitors revealed to me was that my sleep is basically good as long as I pave the way for it. How deep and effective it is, however, depends on several factors:

- When I eat the last meal of the day and how much I eat
- How late and how hard I exercise
- Whether I work in the evening
- Whether I am sick or in good health
- Whether I have to get up early the next day

Having made these discoveries, I make an effort to avoid eating or exercise after 6.00 p.m. I can probably thank my natural constitution for the fact I have worked such long, erratic hours for so many years without falling ill.

When it comes to assessing my sleep phases, I rely mostly on the Oura Ring, which gives a fair indication of the night's sleep quality and recovery. The Garmin watch proved slightly less precise in its assessment of sleep phases but offers a better picture of the quality of recovery.

Lillian (50)
All my life my attitude has been that sleep steals valuable time from my life. Through all my years working and raising children I have been up late burning the midnight oil because that time of night offered good, peaceful moments in contrast to my hectic days. I got used to so little as five or six hours of sleep a night without noticing how little energy I actually had. This became my normal level of functioning.

But now that I have learnt how important it is to get enough sleep and to have a steady circadian rhythm, from listening to my body and using a Garmin watch and an Oura Ring, I have become someone who goes to bed early and sleeps eight to nine hours every night.

Even though I was previously burning the candle at both ends, fortunately I can make better choices in the future and instead have one strong flame on one side!

Your exploration

If your primary struggle is with sleep, I would recommend the Oura Ring. It was specifically designed with the aim of monitoring sleep. In addition to providing a good and precise assessment of the pattern and quality of your sleep, it offers you the opportunity to listen to relaxing soundtracks and meditations. The Oura Ring takes you on a gentle, sleep-inducing walk along the south coast of England. You might in addition use the Garmin watch or a HRV app, to give you greater insight into which of your daytime activities affect your sleep.

Here are some tips on what to test out: first look at the effects of late meals, late exercise, late stress, and alcohol. Concentrate on changing one thing at a time, or you won't know which habit is responsible for any one change. Sleep is central to several sections in this book, and as you find more keys to de-stressing and to increased heart rate variability, your sleep will also improve.

It should be pointed out that your degree of alertness or clarity at the moment of waking is not always a reliable measure of how well you have slept. The exact sleep phase from which you wake also plays a role. Wait an hour and see how clear-headed and rested you feel then.

Try to control your light levels through the day. Expose yourself to outdoor light as early as possible after waking, preferably for 20 minutes. This regulates the sleep-inducing hormone melatonin, which will start to be secreted 12 hours later. Indoor light is too weak to affect the brain centre which controls the circadian rhythm. Remember, the light sensor in your body's biological clock was developed long before the light bulb. Have your morning coffee by the window or, better still, take a leisurely morning walk. Towards evening, you should dim the lights in the house. Listen to an audiobook or podcast rather than staring at a bright screen. Turn your mobile phone or PC onto night mode to avoid the blue light that encourages wakefulness.

Do whatever you can to keep your bedroom completely dark. If you can't, use a sleep mask. This can be particularly useful when travelling, as hotel rooms often have poor curtains or random sources of unwanted light. Try to find out the room temperature in which you sleep best. Most people prefer a temperature of 17–18°C.

Take the time you need to improve your sleep quality before going further in this book. This will help increase your willpower and mental clarity – giving you the best foundation for the next challenge. Remember there's no rush. The important thing is to be patient, and to take a slow but sure approach to introducing new, improved habits.

The monitors I've described use the rhythm of your heartbeat to assess sleep phases. This clearly has certain limitations compared to the measurement of brain activity with an EEG machine. Your monitor may interpret calm breathing as sleep, even if you are just at rest or reading in bed. If precise measurement of sleep phases is important to you, I would recommend the MUSE headband with its EEG meter, which can analyse your brainwaves (www.choosemuse.com).

People who breathe through their mouths experience reduced sleep quality. You will improve your night's sleep significantly by breathing through your nose instead of your mouth. When you breathe through your nose, your body absorbs oxygen with far greater efficiency. The air also contains more nitric oxides, which improve blood circulation and reduce fluid loss, so your mouth gets less parched and irritated. Finally, filtering the air through your nose protects the sensitive alveoli in your lungs against unwanted particles and microbes.

Human beings are designed to breathe through their noses and eat and drink with their mouths. Breathing through the nose during the day – preferably even when you exercise – will make it easier to breathe through your nose at night. If you find this difficult, you can try to close your lips with special sleep tape available from your pharmacy. Put this on half an hour or so before going to sleep. If it feels strange to begin with, test it out gradually – for example during a morning nap. Taping your mouth shut may seem rather extreme, but it can be a simple solution to a big problem.

Note that you can sleep badly and still recover well. My interpretation of this is that good sleep is important for brain recovery and maintenance, while simply being in the parasympathetic resting mode at night is important for recovery and maintenance in the rest of the body. Thus, you can wake up with a foggy brain due to poor sleep, while your body seems fully recovered and ready for action. The opposite can also happen: the body has had a hard time recovering after a strenuous day, but you have slept well.

If you are plagued by unwanted thoughts in the evening, I would suggest one of two things. First, write your thoughts down in a journal before going to bed. You might then be able to set them aside before nightfall. The second one is to write a morning diary and start the new day by putting your thoughts on paper. In the evening, you can then tell yourself that your worries can be left until the morning's writing. Although neither solution is perfect, it's better than letting your thoughts run wild so you don't get any peace.

But what if the data shows poor sleep quality even after you've followed all this advice? In that case, ask your GP to refer you to a sleep clinic. This may reveal an underlying sleep disorder.

Heddy Anne (63)
For many decades I struggled with waking up at night and I have been on a good number of sleeping courses. Nevertheless, time and time again I gave up on trying to sleep through the night and got up around 4.00 a.m. But now that I am able to lie quietly in bed and charge the Body Battery, the problems I have with sleeping stress me out less than they did before. I now understand that I can compensate for lost sleep through resting.

STAGE TWO: STRESS

We are all too busy. We get too little sleep, gorge ourselves on fast food while we are on the go, fill up our tanks with coffee, and wind down with alcohol and sleeping tablets. Stress circulating through our bodies can temporarily infuse us with energy, but over time symptoms such as hyper-activity, aggressiveness, impatience, irritability, anger, self-absorption, and insensitivity towards others will appear. We are not going to stop having stress in our lives; we just need to adjust the amount and intensity of it. Nobody has perfect control over their stress balance. But we can get our stress level to one that we can live with, or, at the very least, take steps to be better than we were before.

It is just as wrong to expend energy without relaxing as it is to relax without expending energy. Too little stress in our lives is just as bad as having too much. The good news is that if you are person who stresses a lot, then even a *little* rest will help you. If you stress too little, then just a *little* effort will have a positive effect.

We are going to explore the degree of intensity and duration that a certain activity imposes on us in terms of stress, and whether the stress becomes balanced through recovery. We will also learn to embrace stress, even if the stress is undesired, because without it we would not be able to develop resilience.

Soon you will find out which everyday activities produce the most stress for you. You are definitely going to make some surprising discoveries.

> **Randi (43)**
> It is surprising what gets the body into a state of rest and what produces stress. An active day at work can provide more recovery for your body than having a day off. Gaining knowledge about what puts stress on our system and what does not is an interesting thing to do.

The science

If you are like me, you may have believed that all stress is bad and to be avoided. Doctors have also thought this for many years. However, science has completely pivoted on this subject. Being stressed can be beneficial for your health! But this is only true if you believe it. It appears that the negative effects on our health caused by worrying about the negative effects of stress may be more harmful than the stress itself.

In fact, there is no such thing as bad stress. Even the stress that we perceive to be very negative offers us the opportunity to grow and become stronger. Human beings were designed to be able to perform under strong resistance. We are descended from people who could do it. Hans Selye, who in the 1950s introduced the concept of stress into the field of endocrinology from industrial terminology, also pointed this out. In our everyday lives, the word 'stress' is used to refer to many different types of burdens including everything from comments on social media to serious illnesses. What people consider to be stress in surveys includes, for example, problems working out a family's schedule, the content of the news in the media, pressure at work, personal relationships, and their state of health. However, stress is not only what we refer to in everyday speech as stress – it is not just a subjective experience. Stress is a measurable set of objective physiological events in the body, which consists of responses in the brain, the hormonal system, the immune system, and a number of inner organs. We can be stressed without being aware of it.

> **Lise (28)**
> I have learnt that watching TV is very stressful for me, so I've stopped doing it. Now I read more books, which is something I have been wanting to do for a long time.

Hans Selye differentiated between negative and positive stress (*eustress*). But for some reason, negative stress is lodged more strongly in our collective memory, while an understanding of the benefits of positive stress vanished.

In the same way that enduring heavy amounts of stress at the gym makes our muscles stronger and improves our physical fitness, the burden of stress can make us stronger mentally and thus increase our resilience. Situations that are forced upon us often offer us the opportunity to grow the most – perhaps because we would never have thought to tackle such an enormous task voluntarily. By overcoming a difficulty, painful as it might be, we become stronger and gain experience we otherwise would not have had. The key lies in how we are able to deal with an obstacle and the solution to this can be found in the way we think about it. According to American psychologist Kelly McGonigal, our perception of stress is the most important factor here. Instead of focusing on the negative aspects of stress we should appreciate its positive sides, and then our physiological and emotional experience of stress would change.

When we are stressed out, our body not only secretes cortisol, but also the neurosteroid DHEA, which strengthens the functioning of our brains. If we view stress positively, the increase of DHEA within ourselves is relatively greater than if we look at it negatively, and this in turn increases our brain's productivity. When our thoughts and feelings relate to a certain activity, our physiology 'listens' to them and changes its response accordingly. So, when we think differently, our physiological response changes and out of this we can then end up having a different result.

Kelly McGonigal distinguishes between a threat response and a challenge response. In a threat response we do not think we will be able to do a task and we get defensive, saying to ourselves: 'I can't handle this; it's too much.' In a challenger mode we do think we can do something, and we go on the offensive, telling ourselves: 'I can handle this; I possess the resources to face this.' In the threat mode our heart rate increases while our smallest veins contract. We have probably inherited this via evolution in order to minimise the amount of blood we would lose if bitten by a predator or injured while fleeing. In the challenger mode, the force in our heartbeat increases while our blood vessels dilate in order to maximise our physical and mental efforts such as during hunting or before giving an important lecture. We have, therefore, a sympathetic, activating nervous system which has been especially developed to mobilise stress. This includes positive stress that is connected to the joy we experience while chasing something as well as negative stress connected to fleeing. Both trigger physiological changes that create new neurotransmitters. These connections enable us to perform better the next time we face a challenging situation.

One obvious disadvantage of sustained stress, both positive and negative, however, is that it can gradually deprive the body of the chance to do some clean-up work and recover after the stress. Even if we are passionate about something, we need some time to rest so that we do not burn out. The positive effect of stress will, in other words, disappear if the amount of stress is too great in relation to our capacity to handle it. It in fact seems as if our body has to be in the parasympathetic mode in order to be able to 'turn on' the recovery process. As long as we manage to balance stress with rest then we can handle periods of stress well. Nature has created us to be able to do this. It is long, unbroken periods of chronic stress that are so harmful. The release of cortisol from the adrenal glands will gradually weaken the immune system's ability to function optimally and that is completely independent of whether the stress is mental or the result of intensive work, a bad diet, alcohol, obesity, or a lack of sleep or exercise. Human beings have one simple biological response to stress – and yet can be subjected to an infinite number of possible stress factors.

Chronic stress leads to a sustained condition where there is an excessively high level of cortisol and chronic inflammation in the body. It results in both psychic and physical symptoms even if the causes are physiological. A traumatic childhood is among the most common causes of chronic, debilitating stress. Most often the traumas are attributed to parents being so physically or mentally absent, unstable, and/or abusive that the children have had to endure a great amount of stress for years. These children have often had to consider everyone else before themselves and so end up carrying this pattern of behaviour over into their adult lives. The stress and hypersensitivity that result from this are often hidden from the person in question – these things often feel like an inherent part of their being and the way they have lived since childhood. Heart rate monitors can reveal the reality of this situation: a hyperactive, constantly switched-on nervous system that is struggling and is wearing down the body. If you think that you belong to this category of people, then I strongly recommend that you read *When the Body Says No* by Gabor Maté.

Thus, the main thrust of this chapter is not that you should remove all stress from your life but that you should learn to spice up your life with positive stress in manageable amounts, and accept that unavoidable negative stress is something you can actually tolerate for periods of time. Perhaps the most important thing to do is to reduce the amount of unnecessary stress.

If your stress level is persistently high and you are not able to get control over it, you should contact a doctor for help.

Recommended reading
The Seven-Day Stress Prescription by Dr Elissa Epel
The Upside of Stress: Why Stress is Good For You (and How to Get Good at It) by Kelly McGonigal

Heddy Anne (63)
Emotional stress affects me much more than making a strenuous physical effort does. Freeing myself from a flood of adrenaline is not easy to do. My body has problems accommodating my attempts at recovery whether it is breathing exercises, meditation, or purely lying down to rest. But after a short, hard workout, my recovery goes much

better. My body has been telling me this for years and now the Body Battery has given me proof of it.

Micro-breaks are also brilliant for me. I have made having them into a habit by lying on the floor with my legs elevated, *without* the telephone on, in between different changes of circumstance such as, for example, between preparing for customers at my home office and leaving to go meet them.

It has never occurred to me that *I* would need anything like this – I'm not timid or weak! But this trick is among the most useful life changes for me.

From the doctor's practice

One of the things that struck me the most during my many years at my practice is the kind of patients who do *not* attend: busy people with packed schedules who do pleasurable work, have a great enthusiasm for what they do, and a lifestyle so all-consuming that it could be quite stressful to maintain in the long run. It is not that I never see them, but it happens far less often than I would have imagined. When they do appear, it is usually because something has become just a little too much for them to handle and they have reached their limit, such as being involved in a project that has gone off the rails or an unexpected, negative incident that has happened in their family. Equally surprising is how rarely they need to increase the number of any subsequent follow-up visits over a longer period of time after their first visit. They gladly take on board advice and they follow it because of their obvious need to return to being active as quickly as they can. They do not consider stress and being busy to be harmful. They are keen on relaxing when they can and make sure that they have activities in their free time that offer them the opportunity to engage in a variety of pastimes. Even though they seldom visit a doctor, I have met enough of them in other contexts in life to know that they exist and that they are flourishing.

It is obvious that people who use more resources than they have will suffer from health issues. Less intuitive to us perhaps is that those who undergo the least stress are the ones who get ill. Patients fall into these two extremes: those who do far too much without stopping to rest and those who do far too little without being active.

The latter group is among those who cope the worst with life even if they tend to have the least stress to deal with. They rarely have things that have to get done with a sense of urgency and little is at stake. They do few very meaningful activities or inspirational activities and rarely experience enthusiasm. When they do not use their capacity to push themselves and utilise their resources, it atrophies like a muscle. They have a low tolerance for stress, are able to endure less and less strain, and lack energy for physical and mental efforts when the need for them arises. They breathe heavily climbing up stairs and let out a deep sigh when facing difficulties. The lack of substance and meaning becomes unbearable for them. A life not lived at all is the saddest thing to see.

We should not relax so much that we become sluggish. Or revel in comfort so much that our lives become uncomfortable. Still, all hope is not lost if you should find that you belong to this group of people. Expose yourself to challenges that stress you but do it gradually.

Malin (37)

I am a social, extroverted person. But nothing drains me of energy more than being social. I've noticed how much worse the Body Battery charges during the night after a day full of socialising, not least when I am among people I don't know. The stress level increases, and the next day I wake up less rested than normal.

Often a downward, negative spiral begins like this: if I have one day that is stressful and drains me of energy, followed by sleeping lightly and poor charging of my energy, it can take days before I feel settled enough to be able to charge properly during the night. And it also happens that during the day when I lie down to relax the Body Battery won't charge. Maybe I am constantly a little stressed out?

At the opposite end of the activity spectrum is another type who struggle: those who appear to be constantly in a frenzy of activity. Their engine runs at a high intensity from morning to night. As soon as they indulge themselves with a little relaxation, this form of 'laziness' quickly gives them a guilty conscience. This approach to life functioned well for them when they were younger, in much the same way that you can get more use out of a newer car than one that has been on the road for many years. But then unexpectedly a difficult additional load of stress appears in their lives – perhaps in the form of contracting glandular fever, going through a break-up, handling a conflict at work, or dealing with the death of a family member – and they find themselves unable to adapt to the demands of the new circumstances. Whereas before they may have been able to handle these things to some extent intellectually or physically, now trying to do so has suddenly become too much for them. Still, they keep plugging ahead, employing even more willpower, expending more energy. Their resting heart rate increases, and the quality of their sleep diminishes all the way up to the day they hit a wall and even the simplest task becomes impossible to do. Maybe they will become bedridden. Often, the whole family suffers.

Once the bubble has burst, it may take them years to recover. Being frustrated and unwilling to accept the new situation drains them of all their energy and prevents them from making a recovery. Often, this leads to a state of inflammation which over the years can result in diseases such as fibromyalgia, fatigue, cancer, oesophageal problems, heart disease, and diabetes. This group of patients are particularly poor at assessing their own stress levels.

So, if you are among those who maintain a very high tempo in your life, I think using a heart rate monitor will be really helpful for you in terms of practising preventative health. Doing this will help you so that you will not end up becoming fatigued, on sick leave, and perhaps on disability benefits, something which often happens to people who live such a stressful life. We need ultra-productive people like yourself to be healthy and in good shape!

Women seem to be over-represented in this group and I meet them daily at my practice. With men in the same situation, six months may pass between their visits. It also seems as if women in general have a greater tendency to take on emotional stress in addition to the stresses of their career and daily life. People who are highly energetic as well as highly sensitive – in other words those who are trying to manage everything while considering others more than they do themselves – are the ones who experience the most harmful states of stress. This combination appears to be more common in women than men.

> **Hanne (52)**
> Since I began keeping track of data with a Garmin watch, I have always been able to recharge pretty well during the night and I usually wake up with the Body Battery between 70 and 100 every morning. But when I went to my cabin, which is 900 metres above sea level, I had bad readings for five days before the levels came down again to normal. I didn't do any other activities than the ones I normally do at home so I must have been reacting to the elevation I was at until I became acclimatised to it.

My exploration

In medical school we only learnt about the negative aspects of the sympathetic nervous system. It was referred to as being an unpleasant, fear-based *fight, flight, or freeze* system which was only triggered by unpleasant experiences. After a childhood affected by being bullied and living in a lot of fear, I learnt to cope with stressful emotions as if I were immune to them. As an adult I have been able to make fearless choices.

As my medical school training inclined me to accept the idea that we entered sympathetic mode only when we were scared and threatened, for years I assumed that, because my life featured more joy than fear, I was in a more or less continuous parasympathetic mode. I was greatly surprised, therefore, when the first results from my monitor appeared on the screen. For the most part, I was in the sympathetic activated mode! Me, someone who has been so fortunate to be able to live a life with the continual freedom to choose both a job and leisure activities that I love doing! My nervous system was firing on all cylinders from morning to evening and even into the small hours of the night. Just as shocking for me was to realise that I could also be in a physiological stress mode when I felt relaxed and was lying on the sofa. Getting into a resting mode after exerting myself took longer than I thought.

I also marvelled at how even less demanding, everyday activities such as socialising with friends, shopping, being in meetings, and talking on the telephone could keep me in a low stress mode. On my Garmin watch, the Body Battery emptied more quickly than bathwater going down a drain. I found out that being focused, playing around, and having fun could be just as demanding as resting after a hard day at work. In fact, the weeks I am away on holiday are some of the most stressful ones! The heat, eating a lot, late meals, leisure activities, unfamiliar beds, jet lag, and drinking alcohol take their toll on one's body budget. I have finally learnt to take these (positive) stresses into account when I sit down to plan my day.

Since childhood I have been shy and reserved in social situations. I got palpitations just from having to introduce myself at a meeting, and speaking to a gathering of people was completely out of the question. The first photography workshops I held felt very uncomfortable for me to do, even if there were only a handful of participants in attendance. I gave several talks during the time I was using the heart rate monitors, and even though it was my choice to hold them, it probably meant that I ended up experiencing a maximum of a negative activation of stress. So even though I may have appeared calm to the audience, the monitor revealed that I was fully sympathetically activated.

Melina (41)
Having a lot of stress over a period of time is incredibly draining. Now I have the opportunity to learn more about what stresses me out, and then I am able to make wiser choices based on this knowledge.

Your exploration

When you want to discover which activities put stress on your system, it is important to get a basic overview first. Is your device happy with your readings or does it warn you against a high stress level? Do not become overwhelmed if you, like myself, discover that your nervous system is operating at full speed for most of the day. Gradually you will gain insight into how you can calm your system down by ensuring that your stress level decreases and becomes more manageable.

Sympathetic activation is important for ensuring you have a balanced nervous system. However, a high stress level will require a correspondingly large effort on your part to get enough rest between activities. I will return to resting techniques at another time. In this stage, you are going to find out exactly what stresses you, how much it does, and for how long.

The most important thing for you is to find a stress balance that is right for you. Using a monitor provides you with an advantage here: although much of what stresses us is common to everyone, what stresses every single one of us, and the degree to which it does, is often down to the individual.

Perhaps you feel as though your time is filled with negative stress that is beyond your control? If this is the case then you, out of everyone reading this book, have the most to gain by trying to achieve a better balance. If you can identify any stress-causing factors that you can reduce or avoid, then by all means do so! The main rule to follow here is to take it one step at a time.

Often, various stress loads will end up being piled up on top of each other. If you, for example, should do a hard workout at 4.00 p.m., and then eat a big dinner with two helpings at 6.00 p.m. before giving a talk at 8.00 p.m., the total stress all together will leave you with a very high stress level. And if you were then to think that you deserve a glass or two of red wine in order to unwind, there is only a tiny chance that you will wake up fully rested for a new day of work the next morning. Perhaps the solution here is to reallocate your resources by making a few small adjustments: have a lighter workout in the morning, have only one portion at dinner, have a good rest before giving the talk, and have a refreshing alcohol-free drink afterwards.

To find out how a certain activity stresses you, it pays to plan your day so that it will be a very calm one – apart from the activity in question – and wait until the stress level is at the same level as it was before the activity, before starting a new one or eating a meal.

Do you have too *little* stress in your life? In that case, you would benefit from 'stepping on the accelerator' and adding some challenging physical or mental activities that offer you the opportunity to grow and develop. Maybe someone in your circle of friends is involved in an activity that you can give a try? Go ahead and give it your all, but make sure to allow time to rest and recover afterwards.

Possessing a certainty and knowledge about the positive aspects of stress can help you face life's challenges. The palpitations that occur in connection to giving a presentation, going on a date, or facing another challenge will sharpen you. Undergoing stress together with its accompanying high heart rate is a part of the body's strategy to prepare human beings for directing their efforts, so stress in and of itself is not something to be afraid of or to suppress. Rather than using mental energy on fighting your heart rate, allow it to work for you.

Be aware of micro-stressors, those small amounts of everyday stress that come during moments when, for example, we constantly check and respond to social media, emails, and reminders on our phone. Even though each small glance at these does not produce a lot of stress on its own, these distracting moments pile up during the day. Try to find some methods for reducing this unnecessary stress. You will get some suggestions for doing this in the chapter on active rest.

And finally, loneliness is a significant factor for causing stress. Try to have several micro meetings during the day and add to them as you go along. Smile to people on the street, give someone working in a shop an extra 'thanks and have a great day!', start a conversation with a co-worker at the water cooler (regardless of whether it is work-related or not), and nod and say hello to people you meet while out going for a walk or a jog.

How you can reduce stress on busy days

- Walk slowly
- Take the lift instead of the stairs
- Do housework at a snail's pace
- Breathe deeply and calmly from time to time. Even micro-breathing breaks lasting 20 seconds are a great help!

Kristin (43)

On Saturday I was at a wedding. There were a lot of people as well as a lot of alcohol. It was a fantastic evening. Normally, I would start cleaning my house relatively early on Sunday – I am not the type of person who wastes a whole day! But I decided to approach this particular Sunday differently and plan some time for rest. I started this off on the sofa and watched a TV series with my youngest son while I ate my only meal of the day. I went for a leisurely walk in the woods. I rounded off the evening by lying in bed and reading the latest draft of *The Pulse Cure* while I breathed calmly through my nose. Today I woke up for the first time with the Body Battery at 100!

STAGE THREE: MOVEMENT AND EXERCISE

Yes, you can literally run away from your problems. Being fit is good medicine for depression. One of the biggest advances in preventative medicine is the knowledge that being in better physical shape significantly increases our chances of improving our mental health and living a longer life. The organ in the body that benefits the most from exercise is the brain. We have descended from individuals whose physical efforts were rewarded with a release of hormones that increase a sense of well-being, improve the immune system, build new blood vessels, and strengthen the synapses between brain cells. Conversely, being sedentary leads to us having chronic inflammation in our bodies. It may be easier to exercise our way to better mental health than it is to talk about it. It is very difficult to get into good mental shape if you are not in good *physical* shape. The investment you put into exercising will drain your body budget on a particular day, but over time this investment will pay off in the form of better heart rate variability, physical stamina, and a surplus of mental energy.

> **Anita (58)**
> The data helped me find the right dosage of activity/exercise, and, not least, how long recovery needs to last before I could do the next one.

The science

Human beings were made to be in motion. Movement is important for the entire body and most of all for the brain. When we use our muscles, substances are released into our blood that strengthen brain synapses. A strong heart, together with good, clean blood vessels that can guarantee a flexible flow of blood, is also extremely important. All the body's organs depend on a strong heart. Every single day the heart and the blood vessels supply every one of the body's trillions of cells with blood that is loaded with oxygen, glucose, and nutrients for the repair and maintenance of cells. At the same time, the blood (as well as the lymph) is supposed to carry away waste substances that have accumulated, such as discarded cellular building blocks, carbon dioxide, and debris from energy metabolism in the cells. The best thing we can do to contribute to the optimal functioning of all of this is to move our bodies and, in this regard, the most effective movements are regular, light ones, such as periodically standing up from a sedentary position. One hour of intense exercise cannot compensate for 23 hours of inactivity. A serious and sobering statistic that we all should let sink into our heads is that only one week sitting still can increase our insulin resistance, and thus the risk of diabetes, by 700%.

In order for our blood to reach all of the cells in our body, we have what are known as *capillaries* to do the job. The body's cells are never more than a tenth of millimetre's distance away from a supply of blood. We have a network of capillaries which, in their total length, stretch more than two times around the Earth! In the smallest passages in the walls of the capillaries there is enough space for only one red blood cell at a time. I like to think that the blood needs a good push to fully arrive at the cells it is supposed to feed and then be pushed back to the heart for another round. Our circulatory system works tirelessly for us as long as we make sure to do our part of the job.

Blood is so fortunate to have a motor like a heart. The lymph is not as lucky. Our muscles have to propel it around the body. And while we have 5 litres of blood in our body, we have 15 litres of lymph fluid. The lymphatic system is the immune system's circulatory system with its lymph vessels and nodes strung out along a network. The clear lymph fluid contains immune cells, hormones, and proteins, and in addition transports waste products from the cells that are too large to pass through the circulatory system. Immune cells patrol throughout all our tissues searching for infections, cancerous growths, and other issues that need to be looked after. The accumulation of lymph in the tissues can greatly contribute to the type of inflammation that can be created through inactivity.

Norwegian studies have shown that elderly people who exercise regularly manage without someone to help them around the house for, on average, 14 years longer than elderly people who do not exercise. This reflects my clinical experience as well. There may be several reasons for this finding. Obviously, muscles increase strength and balance. In addition, they secrete cytokines with every muscular contraction, specifically interleukin-6, which in this context suppresses inflammation (while the interleukin-6 that originates in adipose tissue creates inflammation). Larger muscles also form more insulin receptors, which protects us from becoming insulin resistant. Exercise increases the amount of mitochondria in the cells (mitochondria supplies the cells with energy) and this then leads to the energy metabolism becoming more efficient. Strength training contributes to our bodies functioning more harmoniously, reversing ageing, having better self-esteem, reducing the risk of diabetes, heart disease and stroke, reducing osteoporosis, and reducing stress and anxiety.

Fortunately, even a minimal amount of exercise will reap huge benefits for our health. Even just 30 minutes of moderate movement a day has been shown to be sufficient to gain most of the rewards you can get from exercising. But make sure you get a little winded when you do it. Such light exercise can help you return quickly to the relaxing parasympathetic mode.

Exercise is also excellent for increasing mental resilience and overall mental health. Many people automatically resort to a conversational model of therapy when their mental health deteriorates. However, even though your problems can be put into words, it is by no means certain that you will find the solution in them. Exercise in fact seems to be able to provide just as much of an effect. A good example taken from research in this area is when people who exercise often quickly descend into states of depression or anxiety when they are ordered to stop working out for a period of time. Thus, it is not the case that only the mentally fittest people are the ones working out – the opposite is true. Exercise itself has contributed to making people mentally strong. Researchers have a hard time recruiting people in great shape to participate in tests where they are supposed to stop exercising voluntarily for a longer period of time. They do not want to lay themselves open to the great mental discomfort that will result from taking a break from exercising.

The interaction between the body's musculoskeletal system and its inner organs, including the brain, has evolved over millions of years. Pedometers attached to people from today's hunter-gatherer societies have shown they engage in moderate movement for two to three hours a day (15,000 steps), with some greater efforts thrown in from time to time. The rest of the time they are very relaxed. This is the amount of movement and rest that our physiology has been designed to do, and which we should strive to match. Go ahead and be physically active in nature often, like hunters and gatherers do. It will improve your intestinal flora as well as your immune system.

Physical exercises have long been used to develop mental ruggedness. In hunter-gatherer societies, it is common to go through a rite of passage – a tough, mentally stressful undertaking whose goal is to prepare the youth for the harsh realities of adulthood. If courage and resilience were qualities you could talk your way into having, conversing would be enough. But while talking around the fire after the event might be important for processing the experience, it is undergoing the physical strain of a rite of passage that forms the important foundation for developing mental resilience.

Physical exertion that increases our heart rate and stress level is called a *hormetic activity*. This is a voluntary effort that puts strain on the body and which, in the right dosage and intensity, will stimulate us, make us stronger and healthier, and better prepare us for an even bigger dose of it the next time. Methods such as saunas and ice bathing, or in fact anything that increases our heart rate, will make us more resilient to involuntary stress which may otherwise overwhelm us and give us symptoms of anxiety. Hormetic tools thus create stress – a short-term, safe, regulated, self-imposed stress – that increases our ability to be comfortable in the midst of discomfort.

Warning: it is possible to exercise too much! That hard workout in which you got top fitness scores today will not necessarily guarantee you will enjoy an extended, healthy life. Too much sweating and panting can lead to inflammation, put the immune system on alert, and stress the body. Exercise can also send unconscious signals to the brain. The ancient, reptilian part of the brain looks on and thinks, 'What is going on? She won't stop running! There must be some kind of danger!' Stress hormones will then be secreted to prevent the harm to which the body believes itself to be exposed.

This is where a heart rate monitor comes in extra handy as it shows us how long a body is in stress mode after an activity.

> **Ellen (58)**
> Only leisurely walking keeps me in parasympathetic mode. Anything else stresses me out A LOT. That's why for the most part I have stopped doing demanding exercises and mostly do yoga, qigong, and go on hikes in the woods.

Recommended reading
The Joy of Movement: How Exercise Helps Us Find Happiness, Hope, Connection, and Courage by Kelly McGonigal
Exercised: The Science of Physical Activity, Rest and Health by Daniel Lieberman

From the doctor's practice

In 2016 I held a photography workshop in which we travelled around Ethiopia. During travel preparations for it I tried to form a picture in my mind's eye of the people we would meet there. Photographers such as James Nachtwey and Sebastião Salgado (feel free to take a break from reading and google these names + Ethiopia) have taken portraits of a dignified and proud people, but they were starving, sick, and dying due to being exposed to war and famine. During our trip through what is called Africa's breadbasket, in spite of this situation we met a very vigorous and lively group of people. Out through the bus windows, along deserted stretches of road, we saw Ethiopians jogging on their way to school, work, fetching water, or collecting wood. They looked to be just as relaxed as we are in the West when we nip round the corner to the shop. To me, their movements were somewhere between walking and running.

One evening a group of local dancers put on a show for us that featured an acrobatic, energetic dance that lasted over two hours without a break. In between, from time to time the most agile of us were invited to join in. It did not go so well for us. The problem was not just that we lacked rhythm and grace, but also that we were not able to jump around for more than a few minutes before we had to sit down red-faced and panting. The Ethiopians' washboard abs humiliated the spare tyres around our waists. The experience was a wake-up call. I wondered if that kind of force was inside of us. I had a lot to learn from them! After that experience my view of the physical capacity of human beings would never be the same again.

Once back home at work at my practice, I encountered the opposite of this – people who rarely moved their bodies. They did nothing more than they absolutely had to in order to get to the toilet or in and out of their cars to enter a shop.

Patients very often visit me complaining of chest pain. I ask them if they feel the pain increase when they exert themselves. Many of them have to pause to think about that. They usually cannot remember the last time they did something that increased their heart rate. It is not a coincidence that they have shortness of breath and low heart capacity. When I think back to the runners in Ethiopia, it seems to me that it does not have to be this way for my out-of-breath patients. As a doctor it is sad to witness how many people take poor care of their bodies. It pains me to see the results of inactivity such as thin thighs and legs that stick out from beneath big bellies. Nevertheless, I do not have any problem understanding how easy it is to end up in that situation because I used to belong to that group of people.

Many heart patients think danger is imminent as soon as their heart rate increases. And it is no wonder because in the last century it was normal for doctors to recommend complete rest after someone had a heart attack. Now we know that, on the contrary, it is important to start exercising soon after one. Special programmes are set up for rehabilitation after a heart attack. High intensity exercise is also recommended for elderly people to improve their prospects for being able to continue to live at home as long as possible without the need for someone to assist them in taking care of their bodies or to do small errands for them.

I often advise anxious and depressed patients to exercise. Some people benefit from taking medication and/or going to therapy, but, unfortunately, I am rarely impressed by the results of the efforts of the mental health services sector. I meet patients far more often who believe that increased physical activity causes them to feel better in regard to their mental health than I do patients who attribute their improvement to conversational therapy or medication. Get into good physical shape first and see which symptoms remain. That is my advice – both to you and to myself.

But if you feel overburdened in a particular situation that includes many stress-causing factors, exercising strenuously on top of it may end up being a poor way to solve the situation. Then I would rather recommend that you do brisk walking, or strength training with light weights.

Morten (69)
Doing cardio/interval training enables me to recharge better, not necessarily the same night or the following one, but the effect of it is apparent after three or four days. Just moving (walking and biking normally) does not seem to have the same effect even if the length of my trip might be a long one.

My exploration

This is yet another area where I have to bow my head in shame and make a confession. After I retired as an active kayaker in 1989, I did not exercise at all up until 2014. I had made some feeble attempts at strength training at a gym and maybe went on 10 runs during those 25 years. The reason why I did not do anything is perhaps even more embarrassing. A doctor in the newspapers said that the time you use to exercise does not give you any additional time to live beyond the time you spend doing the workout. In other words, it is a waste of time. And unfortunately, this doctor's calculation went unchallenged. I was certainly not alone in using this as an excuse for not exercising. And most people still move their bodies far too little. Only one in ten Norwegians meet the light recommendation of 150 minutes of moderate movement a week.

The estimation of one hour of exercise equalling one hour of extended life has been shown to be totally incorrect. Several studies indicate that those who exercise with moderate intensity for three hours a week, which corresponds to 8,000 steps a day on average, live about six years longer than people who are inactive. If we unscientifically estimate the life-extending value of movement between the ages of 30 and 80, we get the following calculation:

Exercising 150 hours a year for 50 years is an investment of 8,000 hours. Six years of being alive is 53,000 hours. That results in a surplus of 45,000 hours to live. So, by this reckoning every hour invested in moderate movement will in fact give you 6 to 7 hours of extra life. And although the stock market may possibly be able to give similar returns on an investment during the same period of time, we are talking here about reaping the profits of very healthy living. In my opinion, this currency is much more valuable than money!

As soon as I realised how naïve I had been in choosing not to check the facts for myself, I began doing daily abdominal exercises before I got out of bed, in addition to squats and push-ups every day. Combined with a slimming programme, this was enough for me to have an astonishing rendezvous in the mirror with an old friend: a slim, muscular guy I had not seen since secondary school. Two minutes of strength training exercises daily – 15 minutes a week – was enough to do all that was needed. It was no harder than this. I was embarrassed about how much more time I had spent being irritated over the decline of my body than I had doing something about it. In addition to strength training exercises, gradually I introduced running in place for a minute in between patient visits at the practice.

During the last three years I have used heart rate monitors to assess my workouts. The data has shown me whether I am exercising and straining myself too little or too much. One of the big surprises for me has been seeing how long it takes to recover after doing 100 push-ups or squats. Even though I was lying down on the sofa before and after doing them, it took up to an hour before my heart rate variability was back to my pre-workout level. And after late workouts, the stress could last well into the night and disturb my sleep. Most likely, an accumulation of lactic acid caused the activation of my sympathetic nervous system.

These new discoveries informed me that my training sessions as a young kayaker must have been too strenuous. We happily trained to our maximum capacity every day and we did not have any tools that could tell us that we were overtraining. Today's athletes have an entirely different opportunity for optimising the intensity of their training through the utilisation of heart rate variability and monitors. The best athletes in cardio sports use lactic acid measurements to make sure they stay under this threshold for the most part. That way they can withstand more training.

Gradually, I chose to increase the amount of training I did to two or three workouts a week involving strength and endurance training. I have a rowing machine in my living room, so it is easy for me to get going on a new workout. I do intervals with a relatively high intensity: four minutes of fast rowing followed by three minutes of calm rowing. I repeat this four times. When I jog, I run for half an hour. My strength training lasts for an hour, either while I watch a football match at home or listen to a podcast at the gym. If the Body Battery is low or I have had a stressful day, I drop working out.

As soon as I had discovered that cold or lukewarm showers reduced the inflammation that results from working out, I began to add workouts on otherwise busy days. Over the past few years, I have experimented with a good number of training methods to gauge their effects. While working on this book I chose to try going two months without exercising and then afterwards work out more systematically than I had previously. The period in which I was physically inactive was perhaps the most difficult part of my research into my physiology. I became grumpier and more irritable, and I experienced having less well-being due to not exercising. The scale showed that I had lost four kilos of muscle. After adopting the habit of being passive, it was tough to start working out again, but fortunately I noticed a rapid improvement when I did return, both in my well-being and performance. I am never going back to being inactive again! I have learnt to adjust the time when I exercise and the intensity of it to my individual needs for recovery. I need to stay below the threshold for the release of lactic acid if I want it to have less of an impact on my physiology. (NB not all watches measure lactic acid levels but you can also gauge it by HRV.) I fit in minute-long heart-rate-increasing activities such as running in place or skipping rope during the day, and I make sure that I have at least one rest day between heavy workout days.

> **Synnøve (38)**
> I have always thought that exercising was supposed to give you energy, and that if I felt worn out or tired then a workout would always help. It's amazing how wrong we can be!

Your exploration

Being in good shape is useful not only for being able to go on hikes and walk up a flight of stairs. Our fitness also contributes to our bodies being able at any given time to perform their basic functions with less effort. I usually compare this to a car motor. If you are in bad shape, it is like driving a car with the motor of a moped. The motor has to work at high revs, and even then, you will still not be able to get it to go particularly fast.

What is most important is to establish a minimum level of physical movement. For enacting long-term positive effects on your health, the goal is to get the right amount of exercise. We can also overdose on exercise just like we can on medication or drugs. The amount of exercise that gives you the best strength and level of fitness today can be harmful to your health in the long run. If going through your daily life wears you out, you should be very careful about how you exercise. If you work out too much, you can make a stressed body even more stressed. However, proceed cautiously – some people become *less* stressed from doing exercise. Human beings have different physiologies, and what affects one person negatively may be of help to another one.

It will not take long to begin to reap the benefits of being healthy. Two to three weeks of half an hour of moderate activity a day, five days a week, may be enough for you to reach an acceptable level of fitness. If you are not in shape, start gently. For example, go on a leisurely walk in the woods for 30 minutes and up to an hour and assess if your effort is sufficiently intense by checking how long you need to recover afterwards, i.e. how long it takes after the activity before your heart rate variability is back to the same level as it was before you began. Initially, it should not take more than two to four hours before your heart rate returns to normal, with the caveat that there is no one correct outcome for this. What is important here is that you get accustomed to comparing the effort you made with the degree of measurable stress on your system. If you already exercise a lot, it may be a good idea to check that you are in fact recovering sufficiently. If you do not, your body will not profit as much as it could from the activity. Expect to find a few surprises along the way.

One of the most important markers for assessing your general state of health is your maximum oxygen uptake. This expresses your body's ability to utilise oxygen, which indicates the level of your fitness. You can find scores that represent this on several of the heart rate monitors, which can calculate it when you go out for a quick walk or jog.

Several of the Garmin watches have the outstanding feature of giving you an estimate of how long recovery will take after exercise. The WHOOP band is programmed to suggest that you adjust the intensity of your exercise based on its evaluation of your sleep and recovery. If the Oura Ring registers that the previous day's workout was too strenuous, it suggests that you should have a rest day.

Make sure that the time you exercise does not disturb your sleep at night. If you get up too early to exercise before work, you could miss some important REM sleep. You may recall from the chapter on sleep that this phase enables you to use your memory more productively and helps you to concentrate during the day. If you work out too late at night you risk disturbing sleep onset and reducing the amount of early, deep non-REM sleep. That is when the main portion of growth hormones are secreted which contribute to cell repair and muscle growth. Getting less sleep during this sleep phase can reduce the effects of the workout.

It is wise to adjust the intensity of your workout according to other stresses that are affecting you. Remember that the energy required from your job, daily life, and relationships all come from the same body budget. If you have had a hard day and your Body Battery is running low, it might be a good idea to decrease the intensity of your exercise a notch or two.

Be sure to exercise for both strength and endurance. If you have a sedentary office job, take a few short breaks in which you jog lightly in place once or twice an hour. Do ten squats or ten push-ups. If it is too difficult to do push-ups on the floor, then do them against your desk or the wall. Are you too busy? Doing a little is actually doing a lot. Even running in place for 20 seconds has been shown to be good for your health, and on top of that it increases your concentration for the next hour. Do you really have time not to do something?

Many of those who overload their stress balance are 'good at' exercising regularly and strenuously. They squeeze in time for their late evening workout even if they are busy and tired. However, this can quickly become too much for them to handle. There exists a 'good zone' for exercise measured against the health benefits they produce. According to cardiologist James O'Keefe, we should ideally jog at a slow to moderate pace two to three times a week for a total duration of one to one and half hours. Doing it with increased intensity or for a longer period of time will not benefit our health. Exercise that exceeds ten hours a week can, on the contrary, do us harm and reduce our life expectancy. For example, people who run more than 40 kilometres a week have the same mortality rate as those who do not exercise at all. This is due to a significantly increased risk of calcification of the heart's coronary arteries (the blood vessels that carry oxygen-rich blood to the heart) and of heart rhythm disorders. As previously mentioned, in our natural state as hunters and gatherers we moved moderately for two to three hours a day and the remainder of the time we rested. So, exercise moderately and do it in an amount that is right for you. If you struggle from having a high level of stress, go for a walk and include a few hills along the way. Walking is perhaps the most energy-efficient activity that also affects our health positively. In addition, use the occasion to try out some lighter intensity activities such stretching, tai chi, Tibetan rites, or yoga. These improve our balance, flexibility, and agility. You can exercise more strenuously once your stress balance comes into order.

As your fitness gradually improves, you will be able to notice that your 'standard' heart rate variability increases. This is due to the body being able to maintain its basic functions throughout the day with less effort. You will have strengthened your heart's pumping power and the cells will have gained more mitochondria, which allows them to work more efficiently. You then become like a car with a strong motor that can run at the same speed but at lower revs, and at the same time has the power to accelerate while overtaking other motorists as well as when it climbs hills. If you have a weak 'heart motor', it is as if you are driving a lorry with an average car engine. You have to go at full power just to be able to move forward, even on flat ground and at low speeds.

If you are going to test how much a certain activity affects your body, then you should take it rather easy both before and after exerting yourself.

When your body has returned to the same state it was in before you were engaged in the activity, then you can measure how much stress it put on your physiology. (Here I am referring to the monitors that show you the 24-hour curves such as the Garmin watch.) Also avoid eating during this timeframe because doing so can increase your heart rate and thus affect the data.

An alternative to starting gently is to start with a bang. What about going on a pilgrimage? I have gone on several of them including the Santiago de Compostela and Nidaros pilgrimages. After a month of walking, you will be in good shape, and will have reached a goal. However, start the walk at a calm pace and break it up into shorter stages because you will have to accustom your ligaments, tendons, and muscles to going on a long journey. Plan a rest day for each week. When you come home after reaching your goal, you will have expanded the parameters of what you think you are able to accomplish. You will also have had the time and peace of mind to contemplate your existence and perhaps have solved a few of the issues in your life along the way. Not least, you will be left with all the memories from the encounters you had with fascinating people who shared the same mission as you. And along the way, you will have experienced that, although the path to the goal was long and hard, small steps made one at a time brought you there. Moreover, you may think that the journey itself was the actual goal. I usually say to patients that if you have a small problem, go for a walk. If you have a really big problem, go on a pilgrimage.

A trek such as this is difficult to imagine for all those people who struggle to find the motivation to cross the threshold of their doorway to go outside. If you are one of them, I have a trick you can use. Let others help you get past it! Join a local walking group. Go ahead and get a friend or acquaintance to go along with you, one who you think could use a gentle push, and then you will be helping this person at the same time. We have been created to accomplish things together. In addition to the exercise, you will get pleasure from the hormones that delight in the companionship of others.

Maria (36)
When I work out, my heart rate increases quickly. I have begun to exercise moderately instead of completely exhausting myself. Then I have more energy for the rest of the day.

Starter programme for everyday exercise

Starter programme for fitness

Find a long and slightly steep hill in your local area. Walk or jog lightly up it and then stroll back down again in a leisurely way. If you are not in shape, you can start by doing one round trip the first time. Add one more lap at a time until you reach a number you are satisfied with. Alternatively, you can do one round in half an hour, or you can alternate between walking and running. Feel free to start with one minute of running and add a minute to it every week until you can manage to jog for the entire half an hour.

Get a friend to join you, regardless of whether you live in a city or out in the country and regardless of whether you are in a group or not. It makes jogging easier and more fun to do. Pick three set days during the week in which you jog or walk. Put this it into your weekly schedule!

Use the watch to register whether you are eventually able to go more quickly, or if you manage to do the same round or hill with a lower heart rate. On a number of watches, you will be able to see if your oxygen uptake has improved. This measurement will show you how efficiently your body's cells absorb oxygen.

Along the way, you can listen to a podcast whose information will benefit your health; for a suggestion see page 200.

Feel free and set a goal for yourself to improve your fitness during the next six months and follow along to see what happens to your heart rate variability and the quality of your sleep.

Starter programme for strength
Squats, push-ups, and sit-ups are three exercises that will make your most important muscles strong.

Start by doing 1 of each. On the next day, do 2 of each, and then follow that the next day with doing 3 of each, and so on. When you are able to do 20 of each, then continue doing this same amount. At that point it will take you only a few minutes altogether to complete them. When you have reached this stage and can do this every day, you can be certain that your physical strength is good. Take the time you need to reach this level.

If it is too difficult to do regular push-ups, you can start by placing your knees on the floor or do them standing against a wall.

By doing these exercises you will have covered a good number of your muscles and, in the process, you will have strengthened one of your very most important ones – your heart. Our muscles secrete substances that strengthen our brain synapses.

What about adopting the following rule for yourself: do not brush your teeth in the morning before you have completed this powerful start to your day!

Tore (35)
I have now measured my energy levels using the Body Battery on a Garmin watch for just over six weeks. So far, I have been able to notice that shorter workouts (and low intensity workouts in which my heart rate is low) increase the Body Battery, while longer ones (with a higher heart rate) drain it. This is certainly in line with my own experiences as an athletics instructor and personal trainer.

STAGE FOUR: ACTIVE REST

There was a time when we had natural breaks in our day where nothing much happened. We watched the test card on the TV screen in between programmes. We had neither an iPhone nor Walkman to entertain us while we rode on the bus. Today, we can get news from all over the world and have video calls with people across the globe. Notifications from Facebook, Snapchat, and Instagram ding and break up our concentration. We find ourselves on the frontline of a hard-fought war for our attention, which itself has become an attractive commodity. Our days are inundated with constant doses of micro-stressors, and we therefore have to actively step in to create a space that we can fill with peace and quiet. Otherwise, our body budgets will not increase.

Resting, however, is not for the faint of heart; it requires effort! It is easier to maintain a high level of speed than it is to slow down our physiological velocity. Putting on the brakes is an active action that demands a strong level of concentration and willpower.

Out on the road, it is simply not enough just to ease up on the accelerator to get a car to stop. The same thing applies to stress. We have to try to find the brake, to actively seek out a state of rest.

Find out how your heart rate variability is affected by all these disturbances. We can turn stress into peace of mind!

> **Ellen (58)**
> The most important thing I have learnt from this process is that I'm not relaxing when I think I am. I have to work actively to get my body into the parasympathetic mode.

The science
Dr Audun Myskja puts it so well in his book *Kunsten å finne ro* (*The Art of Finding Peace*). He calls it the 'stovetop burner on 1 syndrome'. It states that many of the people who wear themselves down until they are

ill are unable to unwind and relax fully. Their nervous systems flutter imperceptibly on the lowest flame. Not managing to relax and enter a state of calm wears away at the nervous system. This low-grade wear and tear is often imperceptible and can persist for years before a major stress-inducing incident tips us over. In fact, even a poor diet combined with an excess of exercise, insufficient sleep, and drinking alcohol can be enough to put the stovetop burner on 1. This is true for all of us, even for those of you who do not have that much mental stress in your life.

We need to be good at both up-regulating and down-regulating the state of our nervous system. Do not let your stress level vary uncontrollably in response to outer circumstances as many people do. If you do not turn the 'burner' down all the way to 0, there is a great danger that your body will not manage to activate a 'recovery button'. We have to turn off our inner burner all the way down regularly so that our nervous system gets a sufficient amount of rest so it can function sustainably over time. Do not be surprised if this requires more relaxation and calmness on your part than you believed necessary.

Even if you *feel* like you are resting, it is not certain that you are. We have become so accustomed to the speed at which life hurtles forward today. 'I am only doing what everyone else is doing,' my wife said to me when her stress data went sky-high. The 198 people who tested heart rate monitors during my work on this book have also been surprised by how much stress their everyday lives cause them.

The quickest way to apply the brakes is to use your breath. This is the only part of the autonomic nervous system that we can control consciously. No one can decide to digest their food any faster. No one can order their heartbeat to slow down. What we can do, however, is to calm ourselves by breathing more slowly, or even breathe more quickly if we want to shift into a higher gear. In this we have a very effective tool for regulating our stress levels, a physiological 'lever' that is always accessible to us. How we breathe affects our heart rate variability so we can measure whether we are able to use breathing to enter into a parasympathetic, relaxing mode.

By studying tennis players, sports psychologist Jim Loehr found out that those who performed the best were the ones who had the ability to slow their heart rates down by breathing calmly for the 10 to 15 seconds between the moment a ball is out of play and until the next serve is made. Their heart rate could decrease by up to 15 beats during that short time interval. After a couple of hours of playing, this seemingly insignificant difference was precisely what determined the result of the match. Such techniques can also have a remarkable effect on our regular, everyday work. Even making space for 30 seconds of calm here and there can give us the surplus of energy we need to get through our busy days. One interesting example of this is that when the people of Greece stopped having their siestas, the number of incidences of heart disease rose dramatically throughout the country. Another example is that according to NASA, a co-pilot who takes a 26-minute nap during a long-distance flight increases his or her alertness by 82%.

Conscious strategies for calming down the sympathetic nervous system and activating the parasympathetic nervous system appear to reduce inflammation in the body. Athletes often use several strategies such as taking power naps, having cold showers, and getting lots of sleep to compensate for the efforts they put into training, as well as meditation for lessening performance pressure. These methods can alleviate inflammation, increase the quality of our recovery, and improve our heart rate variability.

People who suffer from chronic inflammation for completely different reasons have also found such down-regulating techniques to be effective.

Tore (35)
The combination of fasting and meditation gets me into the parasympathetic mode quickly. A leisurely stroll out in nature appears to pull me out of sympathetic activation after a long day at work.

> **Lena (59)**
> I learnt that I got less recovery from 20 minutes of meditation than I did from playing 10 minutes of Wordfeud on my phone.

Recommended reading
The Art of Rest: How to Find Respite in the Modern Age by Claudia Hammond
Stillness is the Key: An Ancient Strategy for Modern Life by Ryan Holiday

From the doctor's practice

One of the first things I notice about my patients is whether they have that ability to find inner calm. Often it is apparent as soon as they come through the door. It varies hugely from patient to patient. Take a minute to think about, as you look in your mind's eye over the cast of people who make up your circle of acquaintances, how different people can be. Some radiate peace of mind and others intensity and restlessness.

My experience is that for people to be able to endure serious stress during their long lifetimes without contracting any lifestyle diseases, they have to be good at finding some peace within. For some people this may come to them naturally, maybe because they grew up in a home where there was an atmosphere that embraced relaxation and having a calm demeanour was modelled. For others, living a hectic existence in which everyone is expected to be intense and 'on' all the time is part of their family heritage. There, indulging in rest will get a person labelled 'lazy'. Our innate, personal temperament probably contributes to this equally. Some of us can take off as if we have been shot out of a cannon while others are naturally laidback. One of my big pleasures in being a doctor comes from observing the rich diversity of personalities among the populace.

A great many patients describe their daily lives as being inundated with tasks they have to attend to from the moment they open their eyes in the morning until they close them again at night. The subsequent poor quality of recovery that takes place during the night makes the next day an even tougher one. So, then they have to mobilise even more resources, which they may not have, in order to get through the day. Living like this is rarely compatible with having good health over time.

Eventually the day comes when these people appear at their doctor's practice to get medical help and a note for sick leave. Until recently, my communication with patients has been confined to having conversations about the issue they are dealing with. However, heart rate monitors now provide us with new possibilities. Now we can discuss the data. Naturally, over time I have developed an eagle's eye to detect whether a patient has a heart rate monitor and I ask the ones who have one to get out their phone and show me their stress level. Many of them have an a-ha experience. Few of my patients have been aware of the potential that exists in these monitors.

With the help of a heart rate monitor, we can plan the course of progress that a patient's sick leave will take, not only according to dates on a calendar, but also with regard to the extent of their energy resources. After all, the most important healthcare work happens in between patient consultations. By monitoring our own energy, we can see the warning signs early on and intervene before we reach a point where everything has fallen apart, when it becomes so much more challenging to recover.

Malin (37)

I discovered the benefits of bathing in cold water while at my cabin in the summer. A few minutes in 14°C water brought my stress level down to a minimum. A few deep breaths through my nose and out through my mouth brings me quickly into a normal zone and out of a stressful one.

My exploration

Ha ha! I could hardly stop laughing when I heard about it. The nurses at the EMCC (Emergency Medical Communication Centre) at the Nordland Hospital in Bodø had been on a course to learn how to breathe! That sounded like such a useless and silly thing to spend your time on. I went back to studying ECG waveforms and blood test results. There, I could relate to cold, hard facts that were supposed to be of concern to an intern like myself, thank you very much, not some new age nonsense.

Heart rate monitors have shown that the ladies at the EMCC had the last laugh, however. Because among the things that have the strongest effect on the balance in the autonomic nervous system – that which can be measured and read in our heart rate variability – are breathing exercises, which bring our heart rate into resting mode. The body's maintenance systems appear to use the quality of the breathing as a signal to begin their processes. In the same way that we can smile our way into being happy, we have the ability to breathe in such a way until we feel more serene.

When I first studied my data, I was not only surprised – I was deeply shocked. I imagined that my ability to be easy-going and relaxed when facing life's circumstances was quite solid. My entire life I had been told by friends, family, strangers, and acquaintances, 'You are always so calm, Torkil.' However, my heart rate monitor strongly refuted this notion and showed me only a glimpse of a state that was consistent with inner serenity. Although I externally gave off an aura of calm, and internally I felt as peaceful as I could be, I found completely different results flashing back at me on my monitor. I obviously had a way to go.

My lack of ability for finding inner calm probably stems from having undiagnosed ADHD. ADHD can probably explain why I never had enough patience to have a steady job and why I do best if I am able to constantly switch between being involved in different activities. My attention wanders all the time and I rarely work with the same thing for more than two weeks in a row. My hyperactivity has manifested itself for the most part in the form of turbo-charged thoughts racing through my mind. However, I also experience it as restlessness in my body. Sitting still on a bean bag to write this book has taken the shape of an extreme exercise for me. However, if I am going to continue to make use of my opportunities to live a restless, colourful, vibrant life, and enter old age able-bodied and healthy, then I have to learn how to discover some calm within. I have to find a way to make finding calm part of a stable routine in my daily plans.

Like so many other people, I have great difficulty finding inner calm just by sitting still and being present. Maybe this is why doing photography has always suited me so well. It forces me to focus on something while being intensely present. Imagine my surprise then when I found the opposite of what I believed: photography activates not the parasympathetic system, as I supposed, but the *sympathetic* system. The sympathetic nervous system is famous for being connected to fear, flight, and freeze and other negative states but I found it also to be connected to positive ones like hunting, playing, and other fun activities.

In my search for calm, I had my best results through doing simple breathing exercises and mediation with the Muse 2 headband, which is a neurofeedback instrument which uses brainwaves to help you find inner calm during meditation. I have been good at taking power naps, particularly if I have had a poor night's sleep or have been through a tiring day. I employ the techniques that I use to calm myself down during breaks for a few seconds or minutes and all the way up to half an hour. Each one of the techniques provides me with extra energy to be able to perform well throughout the day.

Occasionally, if my stress builds up or I have had a hard workout, I take a few rest days. Then I move at a snail's pace, just like when I am on holiday and I am wading along the shore. I do stretching exercises instead of push-ups and squats. After a few days such as these I sleep especially well and feel like I am in great shape the next morning, recharged and ready for new challenges.

I have observed that breathing exercises, mindfulness, and meditation affect heart rate variability positively. The exception to this is when I do these activities right after eating dinner or a strenuous workout when the stress on my physiology appears to override the possibility for them having any effect on me. Then it mostly feels like I am swimming upstream without moving one centimetre. If sympathetic activation is triggered by doing common everyday activities – whether they be engaging in enthusiastic conversations or doing lighter tasks such as tidying up or tending a garden, or by the mental stress that occurs while solving a sudoku or crossword puzzle – then it will be easier for me to get into the relaxed, parasympathetic mode when combining them with these techniques.

Ellen (58)
Imagine that something so simple, affordable, and undemanding as breathing exercises can work miracles for the nervous system! Why doesn't the healthcare system talk more about this?

Your exploration

Do you consider relaxation to be a form of laziness? Is it ideal to be going at full strength all day? A striking number of 'energetic' people end up with stress disorders such as a headache, migraines, muscle aches, being burnt out, or fatigue. They do not allow themselves to rest. Do they perhaps need to have permission from their heart rate monitor to be able to unwind and relax? Relaxation is important for us to maintain a productive level of being efficient over time. If you are the type of person who is on the go the entire day, I hope that the use of a monitor will give you the motivation to take a well-deserved rest in the middle of that stressful life of yours. What follows are some good exercises for you to be able to calm your body.

Power nap: Start with what is simplest first, namely a power nap. It should not last more than 25 minutes, but if you are like me, you need a few minutes to fall asleep. Set your alarm clock for 30 minutes. This way you can avoid waking up from a deep sleep, which may be unpleasant and could possibly upset your sleep during the night. If you are not able to fall asleep, at least you will still have got some rest. When you close your eyes, it is a signal to the brain that your surroundings are peaceful. In order to avoid disturbing your sleep at night, it may be useful to have your power nap in the early afternoon, but you can test this out until you find a time that works for you.

Breathing exercises: Pure breathing exercises such as, for example, wave breathing, or *resonant breathing*, may be the most effective for calming down the nervous system. I myself use the Awesome Breathing app, but you can find countless others like it. Several of the tracking watches have their own setup for breathing exercises, and they measure your stress level so you can follow the results of doing the exercises.

The secret of the effect of the exercises lies in breathing slowly with the exhalation lasting slightly longer than the inhalation. My favourite breathing pattern is four seconds inhalation and six seconds exhalation, in through my nose and preferably out through my mouth. This amounts to six breaths per minute, which is half of what we would normally do. But do not get hung up in the counting if doing so disturbs you. You can also use this breathing technique for a minute before entering a situation that you know will be stressful, such as participating in a meeting or giving a talk.

When we breathe calmly, we trick our brain into thinking that everything is OK and that there is no need for it to secrete stress hormones. Remember also from the section on stress that you do not necessarily need to suppress or dislike the feeling of stress. It is a part of the body's strategy to get ready to make an effort and it may require more effort to fight against this feeling than to try to take advantage of it. One minute of calm breathing to take the sting out of the stress may be helpful.

If you manage to do 20 minutes in one stretch, that is fine, but 2 minutes at a time spread out well throughout the day can be just as effective. If you cannot set aside 20 minutes a day, then you probably have a much bigger problem to deal with and you should clear some space in your schedule. Keep in mind that doing activities like these is an investment in creating well-being in the present moment, increased productivity throughout the day, and enjoying more healthy years in the future.

Mindfulness is a technique or method that helps you become more present in the moment. Mindfulness may require somewhat more of your own effort and practice than the simple breathing exercises do. I have experienced that doing photography and going on pilgrimages have made me more present in the moment and attentive to what is going on around me and so put me in a better position to experience natural 'micro-mindfulness moments' throughout the day. Stop what you are doing every once in a while, look around, and spend a few moments on being present; become aware of all the small things around you that you normally overlook. One of the things I have learnt from photography is that at any given time we are surrounded by small miracles that will reveal themselves to us if we were to only notice them. How many different ones can you identify? Use your fingers and run them over three different surfaces and then describe to yourself how they feel. Each and every one of these sensory experiences anchors you in the present moment.

Meditation is another effective form of active relaxation that requires a little instruction, and there are many varieties of it. The Oura Ring has guided meditation sessions and sound sequences featuring rolling waves, forest sounds, and soothing music. You can also measure your stress level with it so that you can see the results of your efforts.

Writing can reduce stress. You do not necessarily need to talk to someone within the framework of therapy – you can start 'talking' to yourself. Journalling can in fact be just as effective as psychotherapy, and has the benefit of being free and available to you at any time. I try to write a little both in the morning and at night. It bookends the day nicely. In the morning ideas often appear that can turn out to be useful during the day. Maybe you need to get some frustration out of your system? Before going to bed it is good to put the day behind you with a few words that summarise the day's experiences. When you close your journal, in a way you put an end to the day. One common characteristic shared by many people who succeed in life is precisely that they write and take notes. Thoughts that swirl around in your head creating trouble for you may look completely different when they have been written down on paper. Good ideas that pop up will disappear in a flash if you do not write them down. My little notebook and pen always lie ready for action in my pocket.

But if you think that all the things mentioned above seem too difficult to carry out, just try the simplest trick of all: lie down on the floor and close your eyes for two minutes.

All these exercises offer a way of gaining some control over our autonomic nervous system. Although it may seem stressful to initiate an exercise for the purpose of getting control, the future reward of having more ready access to a calm mind will be well worth the effort.

Lillian (50)
My body gets into the parasympathetic mode when I am in a cool environment. I go into the house if I have been sitting out in the blazing sun. I lie down in a cool bedroom at night. I take a cold shower after I've been to the beach. I sit lightly dressed in the living room in the morning after I have woken up. Then I am able to relax with a cup of coffee without entering into the sympathetic mode.

Increase your oxygen uptake through nasal breathing

As you might remember, breathing through the nose instead of through the mouth can increase the amount of oxygen that reaches our tissues. In addition, we receive a supply of more nitrogen oxide, which improves the functioning of our brains, and it dilates our blood vessels, which improves our circulation. When we breathe through the nose, we aid our brain cells in communicating to each other, improve the quality of our sleep, and reduce inflammation. Use the active rest periods you have to practise breathing through your nose at the same time!

STAGE FIVE: MEALS AND DIET

The food that we eat has a major impact on the autonomic nervous system and the state of inflammation in the body. The type and amount of food we eat, as well as when we eat it, are all important for balancing our body budget both daily and over a longer period of time.

The process of digesting food, inspecting it for possible infections or other dangerous substances, and then distributing the nutrients to the right places in the body requires a lot of energy and this energy is taken from the body budget. We all need a steady supply of food and therefore it can be useful for us to think about what we eat, when we eat, and how much we eat – not only from a nutritional point of view but also from a physiological one. Perhaps you can also try out one source of physiological calm: *not* eating.

> **Synnøve (38)**
> The stress that results after eating large meals at night was an eye opener for me. This is a rather simple thing to change. I have never liked being a little bit hungry, but now I can see that my body and my head aren't completely in agreement about this.

Some clarifications

In this book's other chapters and passages, there is a large degree of consensus regarding the procedures for improving one's health. There is agreement on the importance of sleep, exercise, balancing stress, and reducing alcohol and tobacco. But for decades we have been disputing what is wise to eat. We discuss calorie counting and nutrients endlessly; at times it can seem like a war is taking place between advocates for the paleo, vegetarian, vegan, keto, and countless other diets. Yet what seems to have been completely ignored is the impact that food has on the state of the autonomic nervous system, either directly (through digestion), indirectly (via the food's impact on the level of inflammation in the body), or in the form of the effect it has on the intestinal flora. We can study this through measuring our heart rate variability.

I should state, however, that even after speaking with several nutritionists, I have yet to find someone who is familiar with the diet's impact on heart rate variability. All my findings in this area, therefore, must be regarded as consisting of a few cautious, investigative steps into completely unchartered territory. Noticing how powerfully diet can affect my own stress levels, however, has made me very curious.

I am by no means an expert when it comes to diet and nutrition.

Although I have read a great deal of literature on the topic and listened to relevant podcasts, I hesitate to write about every nutritional method that is supposed to be healthy. Instead, I have chosen to focus on a variant of a diet that a great many professionals agree to be healthy, a kind of low-carb/flexitarian diet with a minimum of refined or fast-release carbohydrates and ultra-processed food. In this diet, you mainly eat plant-based, 'real' food – the kind a great-grandmother would recognise as being something you can eat. The diet also involves steering clear as much as possible of sugar or flour to avoid a rapid rise in your blood sugar levels, and having meat and fish make up a limited part of the diet. This diet resembles what is known as the Mediterranean diet. While experienced dietitians would certainly be able to point out inaccuracies, I have made an honest attempt to research a diet that is anti-inflammatory, that produces the best results on a monitor, and which can at the same time provide us with the nutrients our body needs. I am aware that this is only one of several ways to eat in a healthy manner.

The science

This section on science is among the longest that appears in the various stages. This reflects how complex the area of diet can be. Possibly, you will encounter words and concepts which are new to you and seem complex. However, the essence of this section is this: try to eat a large proportion of varied fruit and vegetables, preferably in all the colours in the rainbow. Try to eat your meals while it is still light out and within a limited window of ten hours. Try to avoid eating ultra-processed food and food that contains a lot of refined carbohydrates such as white bread, white rice, white pasta, buns, sweets, cakes, biscuits, and cookies, or eat these only every once in a while. Our digestive system is not adapted to processing these foods. Eat until you are satisfied but avoid becoming stuffed. That will just increase the inflammation in your body. Drink water to quench your thirst.

The reason why it is important to eat like this is that our digestion is linked to our immune system. Therefore, eating the wrong diet at the wrong time can increase the degree of inflammation in the body. And nutrient-poor food can inhibit the functioning of cells.

Many diseases, as well as premature deaths, are caused by the food we eat. Estimates vary, but according to several studies a poor diet can shorten your life by up to ten years. Ultra-processed food seems to pose a particularly big problem, i.e. food that has been processed to taste appetising and make you want more, and to have an artificially long shelf life – good for the producers' profit but not for you. Ultra-processed food is often an unfortunate mixture of fat and fast-release carbohydrates in a calorie-dense package. Healthy fibre has been removed to make it easier to freeze, which may be necessary for transportation or storage. The food is energy-dense but nutrient-poor, but it can pack a dopamine kick. The original beneficial animal or plant cells present in the food are ground into a powder that the digestive system is not designed to consume. The food is absorbed too quickly into the intestinal system. In the long run, this will make the bowels function poorly, which will let bacteria enter the blood-stream and create chronic inflammation in the body. Meanwhile the additives that are supposed to hinder food from becoming full of bacteria while it sits on a shelf in a shop will also harm the good bacteria located in the intestines. Thickening agents which regulate the food's consistency can harm the intestinal mucosa. According to nutritional biologist Marit Kolby, ultra-processed food is so thoroughly altered during the industrial production process that the food loses its potential to sustain our health. Examples of ultra-processed food include ready-made meals, frozen dinners, soft drinks, energy drinks, sweets, biscuits, cookies, cake, sugary cereals, ice cream, margarine, and snacks.

Having too many fast-release carbohydrates in our diet is connected to developing insulin resistance. A major symptom of advanced insulin resistance is type 2 diabetes. However, insulin resistance will have harmed your body for 15 to 20 years before a doctor is able to determine a diagnosis of diabetes. Insulin is a hormone that is made in the pancreas. It makes sure that glucose (sugar) in the blood gets into different cells in the body so that they can utilise it when they perform their function.

When we eat a lot of carbohydrate-rich food, our insulin levels spike causing our cells to become overwhelmed. They react by reducing the number of receptors whose task is to allow glucose to enter. They 'cover their ears'. In early human history, people ate very little carbohydrate, so our cells were not designed to handle a diet like today's, in which there is access to a large quantity of refined carbohydrates all year round. Since all cells are dependent upon getting a supply of glucose, insulin resistance lowers the energy supply for all the cells in the body, and the glucose does not enter the cells where it is needed. Instead, it stays where it is not needed – in the bloodstream where it gradually reduces the circulation of the blood throughout the body. So even if the blood is filled with glucose, the cells wind up underperforming due to a lack of fuel, as they can't access it. The functioning of all the organs in the body, including the brain, is thus affected by this condition for years before a diabetes diagnosis is made.

Insulin resistance causes a general state of inflammation in the body and over time leads to the condition of metabolic syndrome, which is a combination of high blood pressure, diabetes, obesity, excess abdominal fat, and harmful cholesterol levels. Metabolic syndrome affects an estimated 1 in 3 adults aged 50 or over in the UK, and the number of people who are in the early stages of it is probably just as high. So, we are talking about nearly 17 million Britons who are at risk. Each of the disorders that are included in the metabolic syndrome pose a risk for other diseases to develop and all together they cause many of the lifestyle diseases we are already familiar with, such as dementia, cancer, and cardiovascular disease. The vast majority of lifestyle diseases are both provoked and worsened by insulin resistance, and yet most patients have no knowledge of this syndrome. Unfortunately this is also true of most doctors.

A low-carb diet, which includes food that contains very little fast-release carbohydrate and a lot of fats and protein, has become very popular. When you eat this type of food, you enter a state in which a lot of ketone bodies are created (a by-product of metabolising fat). Cells can use ketone bodies as fuel. Before, ketones were considered to be metabolic waste. Now it has been determined that they are excellent fuel for all the cells, including brain and muscle cells. Ketones are a signalling chemical that also increase the number of mitochondria (the energy) in the cells, reduce oxidative stress (a kind of rancidification in the body), and regulate inflammation.

An important aspect about real, natural food is that it contributes to the presence of healthy intestinal flora. It is only in the last decade that intestinal flora has been raised from being a topic we avoided to it being recognised as one of the most important factors for the body's immune system. At one stage colonic irrigation was popular. Today, capsules with faeces in them, known as 'crapsules', are all the rage. Before, our knowledge of intestinal bacteria was limited to E. coli but now we know that over 1,500 different species cooperate closely with the body's immune system. If we have a good variety of useful bacteria in our intestines, our body will have less inflammation in it. Incidentally, there are more bacterial cells in our intestines than there are cells in our body. We need them playing on our team!

Both the wrong diet and the widespread use of antibiotics have contributed to destroying intestinal flora. In our Western societies, we tend to have about 30% of the bacterial diversity that hunters and gatherers have in their intestines, and what they have is considered to be optimal. How can we encourage the right bacteria? By eating fibre, vegetables, and fruit. Make use of the entire colour spectrum and look to the rainbow as the ideal to represent the kind and variety of food we should eat. In his book *Spoon-Fed*, doctor and dietitian Tim Spector writes that we should ideally eat 30 different types of plant-based foods during a week.

As mentioned, science does not yet know so much about how food affects the autonomic nervous system. However, many people will quickly discover that the amount of food they eat, as well as the time that they eat their meals, will be reflected in their heart rate variability. Certain types of food will affect you more than they will other people. In that sense, we are all pioneers, and what you are able to find out about the effect of your diet on your nervous system will in fact be ground-breaking.

When you eat, you do not just ingest nutrients, you also trigger the immune system to create a state of temporary inflammation. The mere act of eating a meal provokes a degree of inflammation due to oxidants and free radicals (by-products of energy metabolism in cells) being produced during digestion. For four hours after a meal, the semi-permeable gut wall will allow intestinal bacteria to enter the bloodstream and trigger inflammation. This is normal, and temporary. A meal rich in fibre and phytochemicals (plant-based food) seals the barrier again, and not eating food for an extended period of time strengthens it. A leaky gut worsens and becomes inflammatory-inducing from meals that are calorie-rich and frequent, foods that contain a lot of fructose and fat, particularly saturated fats, and from food intolerances.

> **Annette (38)**
> It surprised me to see how much energy is used to digest food. I try to avoid eating too late at night. It isn't always easy to do, but I have become more aware of it, and I am happy on the days I manage to do it. It really shows up in the data on my watch in the morning. Waking up I am rewarded with having charged the Body Battery much better than on the occasions that I ate late at night.
> I stopped eating breakfast a few months ago. I'm thinking of establishing an eating window during the day so that my body can use energy on something other than just digesting food. I used to snack a lot before, but I stopped doing that after I began using a Garmin watch.

The choice of what we eat is an important one, but perhaps our most important choice is deciding *when* to eat, and not least when we are *not* going to eat. Periodic fasting involves consuming few or no calories a few days in the week, such as the 5:2 diet where for two of the days you consume 800 calories or less. Time-restricted eating means that you eat during a shorter period of the day such as within a period of six to ten hours. Studies of animals and humans have shown that such fasting not only leads to weight loss and a reduction of free radicals in the system, but also improves the regulation of blood sugar and increases resistance against stress. The mechanism behind this is partly unknown, but according to Dr Rangan Chatterjee the advantages of periodic fasting are less inflammation, improved functioning of the mitochondria, a strengthened immune system, improved intestinal flora, a better appetite, and the improved removal of waste products.

> **Tore (35)**
> The data has given me valuable insight into my own physiology and how my body responds to different forms of stress. I was especially surprised that my body enters the resting mode when I fast. Before I thought it was the opposite.

During fasting, the cells get better at removing and repairing damaged molecules. If we keep our organs constantly working to digest food throughout the entire time we are awake during the day, we prevent them from carrying out repairs and doing clean-up work. It is estimated that 10% of our intestinal cells are damaged during a day, and they must either be repaired or destroyed. This requires empty bowels. The process is called *autophagy*, something we are slowly starting to understand the importance of. Autophagy means 'self-devouring'. The cells break down dysfunctional components, dispose of what has been destroyed, and recycle what is still of use. Physical activity and extended breaks from eating stimulate this self-devouring activity. When we eat after fasting, the production of new, healthy immune cells from bone marrow begins. Fasting cycles turn on the switch that renews the immune system.

We must also talk a little about drinking beverages. Even people who avoid drinking sugary drinks and instead choose beverages with artificial sweeteners daily increase the risk of getting metabolic syndrome by over 30% and type 2 diabetes by close to 70%. One of the biggest triggers for insulin resistance and the development of fatty liver is fruit juice, which largely contains fructose. The reason for this is that fructose can only be metabolised in the liver. I have used a blood sugar meter consistently over the course of several weeks and I have registered how a glass of juice, a soft drink, or even a non-alcoholic beer raises my blood sugar level at rocket speed. It is probably because I was already in a state of insulin resistance after several decades of neglecting my diet. Instead drink water, and plenty of it. If you do not drink enough and become dehydrated, this will affect your heart rate variability negatively. Drink fluids equivalent to six glasses a day. The ideal amount is perhaps two and a half litres of liquids during the day, some of which can be in the form of coffee (preferably only until noon or 1.00 p.m.) or tea, if including these helps you to stay motivated to do this. Both coffee and tea on their own can have a positive effect your health.

In a book such as this one, I unfortunately do not have the space to explain everything fully. If you would like to delve deeper into the subject of food and mealtimes, I highly recommend that you read the books suggested below or others listed in the bibliography in the back of the book. You can also listen to the suggested podcast below.

What we should eat: short and to the point

There are very many theories connected to the subject of what we should eat. Perhaps we should just make this simple. Based on the lessons learnt from the oldest and healthiest people in the world, Blue Zone researcher Dan Buettner suggests eating the following: mainly plant-based food with 96% of the diet consisting of vegetables, fruit, whole grains, and legumes. We should eat very little meat and ultra-processed foods and few dairy products as well as foods and drinks with sugar in them. And we should avoid overeating.

Recommended reading
Why We Get Sick: The Hidden Epidemic at the Root of Most Chronic Disease and How to Fight It by Benjamin Bikman
Ultra-Processed People: Why Do We All Eat Stuff That Isn't Food . . . and Why Can't We Stop? by Chris van Tulleken
Metabolical: The Truth about Processed Food and How it Poisons People and the Planet by Dr Robert Lustig
Podcast: *The Doctor's Kitchen Podcast* with Dr Rupy Aujla

From the doctor's practice
Unfortunately, most of the patients I see at my practice have poor eating habits. And when I visit a supermarket, I am struck by the challenges

people face when trying to cultivate a health-conscious diet consisting of little ultra-processed food and few fast-release carbohydrates. The shelves overflow with pasta, rice, and bread products and, as I approach the till, I have to zigzag between all sorts of treats like ice cream, soft drinks, biscuits, cookies, buns, snacks, and countless bags of sweets. In fact, 60% of the food we buy is ultra-processed. As a rule, healthy food is more expensive than ultra-processed food, and since many people shop for dinner on their way home after a hard day at work when their heart rate variability is at its lowest level, their willpower to resist temptation is also low. Any choice has the power to undermine our resistance, and supermarkets know quite well what they are doing when they pull us into one big food labyrinth punctuated with carbohydrates and ultra-processed food traps at the till.

For many people who have to visit a doctor, their problem with their diet is threefold: the food they eat, the food they do not eat, and the absence of a period of time in which they fast.

1. The food they eat contains a lot of fast-release carbohydrates, which can lead to insulin resistance and contracting metabolic syndrome. Consuming ultra-processed food increases the state of inflammation in the body.
2. Their diet lacks a varied selection of fibre, vegetables, and fruit, which provide nutritious food for the body's cells and the vital intestinal bacteria.
3. Eating numerous times from morning to evening, with only a short amount of time in between each meal, disrupts the maintenance work being carried out by the bowels.

> **Monica (46)**
> Sweets in the evening . . . they are worse than a glass of wine! There I was lying down watching TV while I was in the blue [on my Garmin watch]. I had some liquorice and boom . . . right into the orange!

My exploration

Up until three or four years ago I did not know anyone whose diet was worse than mine. Even though I was a doctor, I did not care at all what I put into my body, when I did it, or how much I ate. If I was hungry, I ate whatever was within reach. Food was a necessary evil, something that robbed me of my time if I had to pay it too much attention. When I was a medical student, I would buy a bag of buns and half a litre of Coke and put them in my backpack in the morning. Then I could just stick my hand into it and pull out whatever I found was there when I was hungry. This was ideal for a social guy like myself who did photography, studied film, went backpacking, and studied medicine, since it demanded very little time or thought.

All the hours, days, and weeks that I possibly saved through eating this way have likely been knocked off the other end of my life, because for the next 20 years my diet continued to consist of fast-release carbohydrates and convenience food. The patience I had for preparing food while I was working on call somewhere in rural Norway was, to put it mildly, minimal. And being 20 kilos overweight, I was not exactly a role model for my patients either.

However, at some point, completely by chance, the effect that food had on my heart rate variability and body budget dawned on me. I often work in the beautiful Solund archipelago, at the far end of the Sognefjord. The nursing home in Solund served me a delicious dinner every day. And I had a way of measuring the effects of eating it – my weight went up 2 kilos every week I was working there. I could not continue like that. But the dinner was so good that I did not want to stop having it. My solution was to skip breakfast.

To begin with, going without the first meal of the day was a very unpleasant experience for me. After all, I had been eating breakfast for over 50 years. While my stomach was rumbling and I was rather moody, I expected there to be a bright red curve on my monitor (this is the colour for a high stress level on the Overskudd monitor I was using at the time). I was therefore greatly surprised when I saw that I was in a green zone all the way to lunchtime! And this was the discovery that amazed me the most because it showed me the major impact that food had on the nervous system.

Eventually, I learnt that fasting until lunch made me almost resistant to physiological stress. The initial discomfort – which was probably due to feeling dissatisfied, hungry bacteria, and digestive organs that were used to being unleashed in the morning – began to gradually subside. Today, it is easy for me to fast from 7.00 p.m. to noon the next day. My digestive system gets to rest for 17 hours and doing so has also stabilised my weight. Now I weigh the same as I did when I was 18.

Even though it is difficult to assess the health effects of this over time, it is at least clear to me that the time I eat my meals and the amount that I eat have a big effect on the state of my body budget at a given moment. A large meal can drain me of energy before I am going to give a talk or work out.

After I stopped eating breakfast, the periods spent being in a relaxed state lasted longer. I feel more energetic throughout the day. This was all completely contrary to what I had been told before, that breakfast is the most important meal of the day. In Solund, I also experimented with eating a dinner with dessert at lunchtime and having lunch at dinnertime. That week was maybe the most tiring one I have ever been through. My Garmin watch showed that the Body Battery was emptied at record speed. My consultations with my patients after lunch were like moving through molasses. Going on the treadmill or sitting on the rowing machine at 7.00 p.m. were unbearable ordeals.

My meals and the size of them have influenced what time I exercise and meditate, and in order to improve my sleep I stopped eating a late-night snack. I can no longer bring myself to eat a regular dinner before giving a talk in the evening. And I have learnt that my stress level rises sharply by eating chilli, not enough salad or fish, and a lot of fast-release carbohydrates, particularly ones that combine fats and carbohydrates such as pancakes.

I eventually noticed that I reacted remarkably strongly to carbohydrates, so I went out and got an instrument to measure my blood sugar levels day and night (I used the blood glucose sensor Freestyle Libre). Then I discovered something I had already suspected – that I was at risk for developing diabetes. My blood sugar level, which ideally ought to rise only from 4–5 mmol/L to 8–10 when I eat a meal, could easily exceed

12 when I had a soft drink and ate cake. Just a couple of small pieces of chocolate could send it up to 9. So far brownies hold the record with a blood sugar increase to 15. I took a diagnostic glucose tolerance test at the practice, and it showed that my values were a little over normal and on the threshold for developing pre-diabetes, which is the precursor to diabetes. I can absolutely recommend that you invest in a month's worth of registering your blood sugar level to find out which types of food trigger an increase in it and if you are one of the many people walking around with undiagnosed diabetes or if you are in the early stages of developing it. It is important to act as early as possible to prevent the development of diabetes and metabolic syndrome, both of which can have adverse effects on your health.

In short, this is the diet that works for me: whole foods, healthy fats, and low quantities of carbohydrate in combination with intermittent fasting. I have learnt to fast after feasting and to control when I eat, what I eat, and how much I eat, when before I was indifferent to all this.

Out of sheer curiosity, I wondered if it was possible for me to combine fasting and rest and thereby be in a parasympathetic, relaxed state for a whole day. Could religion, which often includes fasting and resting during the week, be right about this? The results were striking. During a calm day where I ate fewer than 1,000 calories and participated only in calm activities such as reading, breathing exercises, meditation, and stretching, I reached my goal. Now I try to schedule days like that one in between my busy ones if my stress level has risen too high.

Your exploration

Your nervous system may not react as obviously as mine does. I know several people who have experienced little change in their stress levels due to eating meals, perhaps because they were already eating an optimal diet. However, this may also be because their heart rate variability is more pronounced if they are, for example, hypersensitive or allergic to certain types of food. One thing that is absolutely certain is that digestive disorders can cause stress – and stress can be the cause of the disorders. It is particularly important to take into account the impact of the food and meals that you eat in the calculation of your body budget and your accessible energy.

Test whether it may be beneficial for you to finish eating early for the day and then to have a late start the next day. Keep in mind that eating even a small meal, such as an apple, a few nuts, or a piece of chocolate, in fact counts as a meal. The whole digestive system is being awakened at a time when it is designed to rest. It is like starting a car engine just to have it idle for a little while.

As mentioned, when you are trying to assess the effect your meals have on you it is important that you avoid stressful activities that may disturb you during the same period. Feel free to lie on the sofa for an hour before and after eating a meal. This last piece of advice is meant to be followed so you can measure the effect of an individual meal. Physiologically, it may be a good idea to go for a walk before or after eating a meal since your muscles help to metabolise carbohydrates and thus mitigate the increase in your blood sugar level.

Ideally, you and your children should avoid fruit juice. It is full of fructose, which is metabolised only in the liver (and not in all the body's cells as glucose is); too much can cause fatty liver, even in children. Non-alcoholic fatty liver disease is a trigger for insulin resistance and type 2 diabetes. Instead drink water and eat the fruit that the juice comes from, that way your blood sugar level will increase more slowly because you are also ingesting the fibre found in the pulp. Feel free to try the keto diet, a vegetarian diet, or intermittent fasting. What happens when, for example, you eat fewer than 1,000 calories a day? You might follow the advice of the food journalist Michael Pollan: 'Eat food. Not too much. Mostly plants.'

When we use our monitors to evaluate our diet, we find ourselves in unchartered territory. What you can find out from the data can therefore be used for mapping out a new territory. You will almost be like Columbus on his way to America!

Please share what you find at thepulsecure.com.

Recommended reading
The Complete Guide to Fasting: Heal Your Body Through Intermittent, Alternate-Day, and Extended Fasting by Jason Fung with Jimmy Moore
Food Rules: An Eater's Manual by Michael Pollan

Melina (41)

I have been surprised by how much stress has appeared in the data after a meal and how long the stress lasts. Subsequently, I have become better at not eating so late, at being more conscious of eating only when I am hungry, and not to necessarily eat breakfast, lunch, or dinner just because we have been conditioned to do so.

If I am exhausted and my energy is low, I will eat a lighter meal, such as a salad, so that I won't become even more tired like I am after a big meal that has meat in it.

I am not a vegetarian. I mostly eat white meat and chicken. But during the last month, the majority of the days I have eaten mostly vegetarian food and I notice that there is a clear difference in my energy levels. And my body recovers a little more quickly. This is also evident on my watch. On the days in which I need to be a little more on my toes, I have been less hungry. And now I am starting to understand why.

STAGE SIX: THE HIPPO (ALCOHOL)

We have now gone through our Big Five, the stages that represent the biggest challenge to our health. But even if we have tackled the elephant, the lion, the rhinoceros, the leopard and the water buffalo – what about the hippopotamus? It is big but not hard to hunt. Yet supposedly, the hippo is the animal responsible for killing the most humans in Africa, reputedly 500 a year. That is more than all the Big Five put together. Could the hippo's secret perhaps be its ability to keep well-hidden underwater combined with its unpredictable temperament?

Like the hippo, our next challenge, alcohol, may appear threatening in a rather strange way. It is unusual for people not to drink alcohol. When I say no thank you to a beer or a drink, people look at me suspiciously as if to say, 'What is wrong with you? Why on Earth don't you drink?' And maybe it is not so surprising that abstaining causes such a stir: only one in ten Norwegians refrain from drinking alcohol completely.

Another one in ten Norwegians drink in such a way that risks leading to addiction and harming their health. Between these two extremes you will find 80% of the people who drink within the limits of what is considered socially acceptable. However, these people too pay the price physiologically for drinking. If you drink alcohol and at the same time measure the impact of it on your monitor, you have probably already discovered the effect it has.

Even though it is well known that high alcohol consumption disposes us to several different diseases, we know little about the impact of alcohol on how we function in everyday life. It is striking that 80% of those who use the WHOOP fitness tracker have cut down their alcohol consumption on their own initiative after seeing the effect of alcohol on their sleep and stress. You can expect more such surprises to appear in the pages ahead.

In this section I am not going to talk about alcoholism. I am going to confine myself to what is considered normal consumption, i.e. the recommended limit of 14 alcohol units a week, which is often not thought of as posing a problem to our health.

If alcoholism is a problem for you or your loved ones, contact your doctor, or Alcoholics Anonymous. Their 12-step programme has helped many people escape the clutches of alcohol.

Synnøve (38)
In my hectic everyday life, it used to feel as if enjoying a small glass or two of wine at night gave me energy. The fact that it is expensive or unhealthy did not stop me or my husband from drinking. But seeing the toll that a glass of wine takes on the Body Battery gave us a solid reason to reassess what we were filling our glasses with.

The science

The earliest evidence that people drank alcohol goes as far back as 13,000 years, to Haifa in Israel. The alcohol was probably used in religious rituals. In fact, having regular, consistent access to alcohol may have been a factor behind motivating human beings to become farmers.

Today, alcohol consumption is widespread. About 35% of Norwegians drink it weekly. Abstinence is in fact more common in Italy and Portugal where up to 30% of the population never drink alcohol. The number of people who drank until they became inebriated during the last year was 60% in Norway and under 10% in Italy and Portugal. In the UK alcohol harm costs society between £27 and £52 billion every year. Within this, the cost to public health and care services is estimated (conservatively) at £3.2 billion, and £7.3 billion is attributed to lost productivity, absenteeism and accidents at work.

Alcohol affects the brain by passing through the blood-brain barrier and 'anaesthetising' the brain cells. This numbing begins in the most advanced parts of the brain and moves gradually down to the autonomic nervous system. The first thing that happens is a degeneration of the ability to think critically. By the time the ambulance arrives because being inebriated has rendered you unconscious, only your heart rate and breathing signal that there is still life inside you. At this stage you are as sedated as if you were just about to be operated on. Over the years, at night inside an ambulance, I have gripped a number of inebriated, passed-out youths hard on their arms without getting a pain response back. So, what is it about alcohol that makes it have such a profound impact on our physiology?

Alcohol is processed in the liver by an enzyme that converts the alcohol into the highly toxic substance acetaldehyde. This substance gives us the unpleasant intoxication symptoms that we call a hangover. We enjoy being inebriated but the toxic effects of drinking hammer away at our body while we sleep. We may wake up and think that we are a little tired, but truth is our bodies have been through an all-night stress marathon. We have come across the subject of inflammation several times already in this book; research has shown that alcohol increases the level of cytokines – inflammatory substances – in the blood. It is no wonder that we feel hungover after we have been out partying. We are, simply, sick. Our body works tirelessly through the night to convert the toxic acetaldehyde into acetic acid, which can then be excreted in our urine. This detoxification process is prioritised by the body to such a degree that it can take a heavy toll on the body's energy, using up reserves that could otherwise be used for recovery in other areas. The worse the hangover, the greater the inflammation. If you drink too much one day, you will in fact become susceptible to contracting infections and illnesses for days afterwards. For those people who exercise, their capacity to recover from exertion will plummet and they will derive fewer benefits from their workouts.

A further complication is the reduction in the quality of our sleep following alcohol intake. Sleeping poorly in combination with the body undergoing detoxification throughout the night is probably the reason why we wake up the next day after drinking feeling more tired than from any other activity. Just two or three innocent glasses of wine can shatter the night's recovery process more than any other factor. As you can probably imagine, your monitor will be able to back this up.

In terms of our health, this is perhaps the biggest problem associated with drinking alcohol. Alcohol is not just slightly disruptive to our sleep, it is disastrous. Even if, the following day, our blood alcohol level falls back under the legal limit of 80 milligrams of alcohol per 100 millilitres of blood our ability to concentrate will still be poor. And as we have seen, over time, poor sleep is one of the most destructive factors for our health both mentally and physically.

What is the cause of alcohol-induced poor sleep? Often, the monitors show a lowered stress level just after alcohol consumption. When we drink alcohol, substances (GABA) are secreted that trigger receptors in the brain which have a calming effect on us. But as the detoxification process begins and the sedative effect wears off, both the heart rate and the inflammation in the body increase. Perhaps this hinders the brain from being sufficiently tranquil for the positive sleep cycles to begin. And perhaps the sympathetic-driven overactivation of the nervous system is responsible for wearing down the body during the night.

In a study of athletes by WHOOP, those who marked that they consume alcohol experienced significant results. Their resting heart rate during the night was on average 15% above normal and their heart rate variability was reduced by 20%. It was almost as if they had run a marathon in their sleep. It took four to five days until the quality of their recovery was back to normal. For them, the impact they felt during the night was more like they were anaesthetised than they were asleep. We may fall asleep more easily from drinking alcohol, but our sleep is much worse.

Periodic atrial fibrillation is a common condition. The heart beats unevenly and the effect of its cardiac output is reduced by 10–30%. Alcohol increases the risk of a steady heartbeat turning into an erratic, ineffective atrial fibrillation. In addition, the risk of blood clots going to the brain increases. This gives us an indication as to alcohol's effect on the functioning of the heart. What is most important for us in this context is that we have received a warning about how strongly alcohol can affect our two most important organs – the heart and the brain.

People who drink a lot of alcohol also have an increased risk of contracting infectious diseases, take longer to heal from illness, and go through more complications due to surgery.

> **Therese (42)**
> I found out that alcohol has a very negative effect on my body. Even if I only drink half a glass of wine in the evening, my body remains in a stress mode throughout the night. That's why I have almost completely stopped drinking.

Recommended reading
The Sober Revolution: Women Calling Time on Wine O'Clock by Sara Turner and Lucy Rocca

From the doctor's practice

A doctor quickly gets accustomed to being rewarded for paying close attention to the external appearance of his or her patients. A lot of telling information can be found in a patient's appearance and the way they express themselves. Just catching one small glimpse of them as they walk through the door may be enough. What goes on inside someone's body and soul is often visible on the outside – at least to a trained eye, preferably aided by a patient's medical records in which one's suspicions of alcoholism may be confirmed. Few diseases reveal themselves as obviously on the skin, in the eyes, and in our general appearance as excessive alcohol consumption. And even for those of us who stay within acceptable normal consumption, there is very rarely any doubt about when we look our worst – the day after a genuine bender.

When looking at town drunks, it is obvious to see that their excessive alcohol consumption is sending them to an early grave. Much more difficult to identify are the people whose consumption is of the less extreme variety. Until heart rate monitors came on the scene, it was difficult for doctors to assess the health effects of alcohol on people's everyday life. Now that more and more people are using heart rate monitors, however, I can show patients on their own mobile phones how their alcohol intake for the week affects the energy they have at their disposal. Athletes who monitor their heart rate variability have for the most part stopped drinking. WHOOP, for example, followed an NFL team (American football) that used to drink together after games. The players quickly stopped when the data revealed how strongly the effect of alcohol reduced their capacity to recover from the game, which could take as much as four days.

Imbibing non-alcoholic drinks has fortunately become more commonplace and less stigmatised. In Norway, sales of non-alcoholic alternatives at the state-owned liquor stores, as well non-alcoholic beers in the shops, have grown considerably.

Heddy Anne (63)
Gaining knowledge about how alcohol stresses the nervous system has been a shocking, eye-opening experience. The idea that one glass of red wine a day is good for your health is obviously false.

My exploration

Again, it is time for me to return to the confession booth. When I was a student, my classmates and I often drank two or three pints of beer together several times a week. Then my student loan formed a natural curb on my spending, but as I became a doctor and did not need to follow the balance in my bank account like a hawk, my alcohol consumption increased. And when some soft news in the newspapers declared that it was ideal for men to drink two glasses of wine a day, I gladly followed their advice!

Most of the time it was quite pleasant to drink those two glasses of wine. It was so pleasant that I ended up getting quite tired and just slept like a log. Or so I thought. When I always woke up in the morning feeling sluggish, I considered it to be normal.

The only nights I did not drink were the ones I was on the night shift. So, I lacked a good baseline for making comparisons. Alcohol functioned for me as a kind of shortcut to a relaxed state after busy, eventful days. This short-cut turned out to have a few stumbling blocks. My data shows that it takes going through a fairly busy night shift before my nervous system becomes as heavily stressed as it is after drinking just two or three glasses of wine.

The turning point came after I had started working at Sykkylven Hospital in 2013. I was on A&E duty eight days and nights (24-hour shifts) in a row and then I had one day off before the next six-day period of being on duty 24/7 would begin again. On that day off, I happily slept in, went on a hike for two hours, and then popped into the liquor store for a well-deserved bottle of wine. After a few periods of work such as this I noticed a pattern. I was much more tired after the day off spent drinking a bottle of wine than I was after being on constant duty for eight consecutive days. Something was seriously wrong with this situation. My job required that I work to my max-imum capacity, yet it was not work that was depleting my energy. I had thought that I only became sleepy from drinking alcohol, but I began to realise that I was subjecting myself to something closer to a nocturnal, bodily earthquake. I, who was so fond of having a glass of wine, realised that I had no other choice but to cut out drinking completely. This was much easier for me to do than having to constantly calculate when and how much I could drink. As I have mentioned, such continual choices cost us some willpower.

I stayed away from alcohol completely in the years that followed.

However, a year ago, when I was going to write a medical paper about my findings from using a heart rate monitor, I thought I should have a few glasses of wine in the name of science. What a great excuse! My findings clearly showed that what I experienced on my day off in Sykkylven could be demonstrated via concrete data. While I slept, my monitor kept watch over me. After three or four glasses of wine, my recovery during the night after was miserable, just out-and-out disastrous.

I also tested the effects of drinking just two glasses with almost equally disappointing results. In fact, no other factors, apart from a severe febrile illness, have caused such a devastating effect on my capacity to recover. The day after I was pretty much out of it. My heart rate monitor's warning lights blinked, my WHOOP band showed I was in the red, my Garmin's Body Battery had not charged during the night and the Oura Ring warned me that I should have a very quiet day. This was a proper reality check. Now that I was aware of what my normal level of capacity for activity was, it felt even worse to go at half speed. The pleasure of drinking is now offset even more by the price I have to pay the next day.

Now I think twice before I have a drink. Do I have the energy in reserve to drink alcohol? Is the fun I get from doing it worth it? It rarely is. I now know that I cannot expect much from myself the day after drinking. Why did it take me 25 years of consuming alcohol to realise this? Perhaps because I lacked the motivation to look into it – I did not want to know – and heart rate variability monitors did not yet exist to show me the effects so clearly and understandably.

> **Maria (36)**
> I am shocked at how little alcohol it takes to affect my body. I was in the orange the whole night after only two units.

Your exploration
The most important reason for measuring your heart rate variability is not necessarily to cut out alcohol completely; it is to understand the effect that

alcohol has on you. The more you understand how it affects you, the easier you will find it to decide how often – and how much – you should drink. People react differently to it. Perhaps alcohol consumption will affect you minimally. Or maybe it will be the opposite, and you will feel its effects more heavily than others do.

Our bodies' responses may also be related to who we drink with and the circumstances surrounding it.

Do you react differently to wine, beer, or spirits? According to WHOOP, clear alcohol has less of an effect on our heart rate variability. In chemist Alexander Sandtorv's book *Fylla har skylda* (*Blame It on Being Drunk*), drinks are sorted according to their decreasing ability to cause a hangover and inflammation: brandy, red wine, rum, whisky, white wine, gin, and vodka. It is probably not without reason that patients who drink a bottle of spirits a day tell me that they prefer vodka.

Try to become familiar with how alcohol affects your body. That way you will more easily be able to assess beforehand whether the fun you have from drinking will outweigh the cost of doing it. Heart rate variability monitors have made it much easier to calculate what the physiological bill will be for yesterday's consumption. Studying these figures is a little like checking your wallet after going bar-hopping and being stunned that the three glasses of wine you had yesterday cost ten times what you expected them to.

With your monitor you will be more capable of judging how much stress on your system you will be able to tolerate the day after a night out. Drinking alcohol affects your concentration, alertness, and willpower the next day. This is not an optimal situation if you have an important exam to study for, a delicate family situation to take care of, or a big hike planned. After a fiesta, the best thing to do is have a siesta.

Anita (58)
When I saw how much two glasses of wine cost me in terms of high stress numbers, poor quality of sleep, and a low Body Battery, it suddenly wasn't so much fun to do any more – and it was relatively easy for me to stop doing it.

How you can test the effects of alcohol on your physiology

If you rarely drink: Test yourself by drinking two to three units of alcohol on a normal weekday at home and do it a while after eating a meal as your stress level will have stabilised by then. If you drink in connection with a social occasion, it may be that the stress that appears on your monitor is not due to the alcohol but to your involvement in the event or the circumstances surrounding it.

If you drink regularly: Keep a close eye on the effects of alcohol the day after drinking during the test period. Try to isolate your alcohol consumption so that the data is not disturbed by other activities. For example, test one week in which you drink alcohol and one week in which you do not. What do you think your results would be if you tried going a whole month without drinking?

STAGE SEVEN: ILLNESS AND DISEASE

One of the most important things you can do to maintain good health is to reduce stress on yourself when you are ill. Acute illness as well as the worsening of a chronic illness can make a big dent in the body budget. Energy that would otherwise have been used for daily tasks has to be reallocated to the job that the immune system needs to do. Many people try to mobilise energy they do not have to compensate for their reduced capacity to function. This is like getting a credit card loan to cover an unexpected car repair. And the longer you wait to repay the credit card debt, the more expensive it will end up being.

A person who is barely maintaining a state of physiological equilibrium can be tipped over into a state of imbalance by an acute illness. The illness is often triggered by a prolonged period of stress with its attendant overburdening of the physiology and resulting poor state of the immune system, as well as inflammation. Unfortunately, I have seen all too many people who need long periods of sick leave due to chronic fatigue, some of whom eventually end up receiving disability benefits.

Fortunately, a heart rate monitor can alert us as soon as an acute illness begins or when a chronic illness is starting to worsen. At that point we are then able to see what needs to be done in terms of getting extra sleep and recovery so that a patient does not become completely drained of his or her energy. If we do not take the illness into account, we increase the risk of the patient continually contracting new secondary diseases. As soon as the immune system is occupied on one front, other diseases launch an attack on another. The list of the patient's diagnoses just ends up getting longer and longer.

What I have experienced at my practice is that certain patient groups experience an accumulation of diseases. The ones who are particularly vulnerable are those patients who are unable to adjust their activities to their capacity.

> **Melina (41)**
> I've been through a few days where I didn't properly recharge during the night and my body was in a state of stress.
>
> My general condition deteriorated slightly, but not to the degree where the results on my watch made any sense. So, I really wondered what could be going on. Was I getting sick? Had I got a new variant of Covid?
>
> It wasn't until a few days had passed that I recognised that I had the symptoms of a urinary tract infection, and I got it confirmed by my doctor.

The science

What follows is a little repetition from the introduction about the *innate* and the *adaptive* immune systems. This is so important that it bears repeating!

The first thing we tend to notice when we are ill is not the illness itself but the symptoms that result from the *innate* immune system's reaction to it, such as a fever, pain, fatigue, lack of appetite, nausea, and a need to be alone and lie still. In the event of acute illness, our advanced, precise, energy-demanding, and slower-to-respond *adaptive* immune system becomes mobilised.

As you may remember, our innate immune system is fast-acting but primitive with a poor long-term memory. This immune system can also be activated by feeling angry, worrying, experiencing loneliness, or doing intense, frantic activities, or exercising. In earlier times, these thoughts and behaviours were often followed by becoming injured and a subsequent risk of infection, so, our immune system is mobilising itself in advance of the expected challenges we may face.

Macrophages are the foot soldiers of the innate immune system. They are immune cells that are supposed to detect and disarm threats that come in the form of injuries and infections. The word 'macrophage' means 'big eater'. These foot soldiers envelop and digest dead cells, foreign bodies, microbes, and cancer cells. They are in a kind of dormant state throughout the body but can suddenly wake up in case of inflammation and secrete substances that will rouse all the other macrophages in the area and send alarm signals to the bone marrow and the brain that the defences need to be mobilised. Macrophages spew out inflammatory substances – cytokines – which are carried throughout the body in the blood, and this leads us to experience what can be called 'sickness behaviour' in which we withdraw, lose our appetite, sleep poorly, become lethargic, feel depressed, and become anxious.

This sequence of responses represents an ancient strategy designed to ensure our survival, both individually and for the tribe as a whole. This freed the sick person from participating in the strenuous work of the tribe, allowing them to convalesce so that the person's resources could be redistributed to his or her immune system. With their appetite having been reduced, less energy was used to digest food. Their disrupted sleeping pattern could make them more alert at night, which could be useful for them because everyone who withdrew socially and found themselves on the fringes of the tribe were more vulnerable to attack. And for the tribe, it was advantageous to put a sick person in isolation because they may have been carrying an infectious bacteria or virus.

So-called sickness behaviours can also be considered as a kind of defeat response. Like many other mammals, humans withdraw as soon as they feel they are a burden to the tribe. Inherited responses like this may provide part of the explanation as to why modern people so readily isolate themselves when they are depressed or not feeling well in general. They may feel worthless and think that everyone else is able to do a lot better without them both now and forever.

The fact that depressed people tend to isolate themselves can partly be attributed to the built-in defeat response, which itself is linked to an inflammatory state in the body. Sickness behaviours can arise regardless of the cause of the inflammation. Research has shown that the presence of cytokines leads to these symptoms. When healthy animals are injected with cytokines, they display the same behavioural patterns as they would if they were sick.

Our urge to stay away from people who show outward signs of fatigue and illness may also be an inherited characteristic, a kind of intuitive reaction. Equally, this stigmatisation could further exacerbate the discomfort of being ill. This is one more component in an illness's downward spiral. And, as in so many other areas, this is another way that our nervous system, which was developed in response to the world of our ancestors, sticks its foot out and trips us up.

One of the most energy-demanding things a human can go through is experiencing a powerful reaction from their immune system. It takes a heavy toll on our body budget. One of the things that is immediately affected is our heart rate variability. The increased blood circulation and activation of the sympathetic nervous system make our heart rate variability sink. Often, it will react before we are able to notice the symptoms. If you were to choose to use your energy on working or other activities, there would be little left over to fight the illness.

Over time, heart rate variability is also an indicator of how great a risk we in fact have of contracting an acute or chronic disease. During a period in which our heart rate variability is lower due to physiological stress, the immune system will be weakened so the risk of falling ill is greater than normal. We have probably experienced getting a cold after going through a stressful period. And as soon as we are struck by it, our heart rate variability will worsen even further.

A constantly low heart rate variability is linked to the risk of contracting nine of the ten deadliest diseases, physical as well as mental, in the Western world. Depression increases the risk of heart disease, cancer, and other chronic diseases – and chronic diseases increase the risk of depression. The previously mentioned diseases are inflammatory diseases that play off each other negatively. This may explain why a number of diseases are able to accumulate in some patients. Heart rate monitoring data helps alert us to the beginnings of this downward spiral so that we can take measures to mitigate the inflammation. Or, put more precisely, put into practice methods that can diminish burdensome stress as well as resting techniques that bring us relief.

Ellen (58)
I try to avoid doing activities in the evening several days in a row. Doing this often causes me to sleep poorly, have migraines, and have a low Body Battery.

From the doctor's practice

As I have spent most of my professional career working as a locum GP and A&E emergency physician, I have chiefly encountered acute illnesses. Fortunately, calculating CRP – C-Reactive Protein – values had already begun when I graduated from medical school. CRP is a blood test that indirectly measures cytokine levels in the blood and shows the degree of infection or inflammation in the body. CRP is the most important blood test you can get in the emergency room. It can tell you a lot about how an illness is developing. I often use it as a precise biomarker for the diagnosis and assessment of the level of infection. Heart rate monitors and HRV (heart rate variability) have provided us with yet another new, useful parameter.

'Which watch are you wearing on your wrist?' I ask patients this question increasingly often. About two million Norwegians have acquired heart rate monitors. In the case of acute illness, when the patient and I look at their smartphone together and compare their heart rate variability with their normal state, it can tell me a lot about how affected that person is by their illness.

Data results are particularly useful in the case of infections that cause discomfort long after the fever is past. One example of this is glandular fever. Covid-19 also has the potential to knock a patient out over a long period of time (*Long Covid*). In that instance, it may be difficult for both a doctor and a patient to assess the prognosis.

With heart rate monitors, I can more easily see if and when a patient is ready to work or to exercise. When a patient has tried to partially return to work, I can see from the data whether their body has handled it well or not.

The data on the heart rate monitor also makes it easier for the patient to show the doctor whether it is necessary to extend their sick leave. It may appear that we doctors unfortunately show more empathy and understanding towards a patient when we have a test result that confirms a disease. Many patients tell me that they struggle with trying to be taken seriously when it appears as if there is no detectable or perceivable cause for their ailments.

Conditions other than infectious diseases, such as fractures, sprains, and operations, will also have an impact on heart rate variability and the secretion of cytokines. These conditions can also cause some patients to withdraw. Even root canals and tooth extractions can cause someone to be completely put out of action, feel sick, experience poor quality of sleep, lose their appetite, and become noticeably unsocial.

Even when you are sick, you should get up and move around a little. After all, your blood has to be propelled throughout your body. The same applies to lymphatic fluid. And even if your fever and the subsequent increased heart rate help to speed up your blood, you can certainly give it a helping hand. So, shuffle around the house a few times during the day.

As in so many other areas, my experience is that the sickest people reside at the extremes: those who pay extra attention to illnesses and have become inordinately passive, and those who give the least amount of consideration towards illness and go at full speed, right up until their body says it has had enough and gives up.

During an acute, severe, short-term illness, it is important to relax as much as possible. If you have a somewhat milder but more long-term illness, you have to try to find a good balance between being active and resting. Too much rest can weaken your body more than is necessary. Exerting yourself too much can set your recovery back. Fortunately, a good balance between activity and rest has become easier to establish since heart rate monitors came on the market. Now that we can concretely see how closely a patient's stress levels reflect the illness, both myself as a doctor and you as a patient have the opportunity to balance your level of activity in a much more stable way.

A deep sigh of concern here at the end: I have often found it very frustrating working in a healthcare system where there are almost watertight bulkheads between the psychiatric and the somatic fields of medicine. Most diseases in both of these fields are characterised by having a chronic state of inflammation which we should treat collaboratively.

> **Annette (35)**
> It was very interesting to see on my watch that something happened to my body in the days before I tested positive for Covid. Imagine, it showed up on my Oura Ring before I had noticed any symptoms! It was incredible how my body worked with all cylinders firing – even though I was lying there in bed without doing anything at all.

My exploration

Once again it is time for me to return and place my head in the pillory. As a doctor I found it far too easy to go to work when I was feeling under the weather, and I returned as quickly as I could after an illness. This is probably true for most doctors. Our profession goes on sick leave far less frequently than those in comparable occupations. Both we ourselves and the society around us seem to expect more from doctors than from other people.

Now, during periods of being sick, I have become better at adjusting my level of activity in the form of resting and taking power naps, and I reduce all other stresses in my life to a minimum. When it comes to exercise, I am more patient than I was before. Only when the monitor tells me I am fully recovered do I start working out again. When I was afflicted with Covid, my monitors were in 'alarm mode' for days in which they warned me not to exercise. For several months afterwards, the monitors indicated that I was struggling much more than I normally did in finishing the walks my body is used to going on.

Although many athletes have said that it is OK to train as long as you do not have a fever, I doubt whether they recover sufficiently after an illness to get the full benefit of the workout itself. The body should probably content itself with prioritising fighting illness and put the repair of muscles on hold.

In fact, since changing my lifestyle, I have fallen ill from respiratory infections much less frequently than before. In fact, the one time I had Covid was the only instance of illness I have had in almost three years. So, it feels particularly good to know that this is the same immune system that is going to protect me against heart disease, cancer, and other serious diseases in the years ahead.

Ingvild (52)
Quite recently I introduced a friend to Garmin watches and the Body Battery. At first she recovered really badly as demonstrated by her low Body Battery numbers (it was at 5 half the night before it charged up to the 20s). Even after getting tips and advice about changes that can help, the effect had been minimal. But then something happened last night – she forgot to take her blood pressure medication. And BOOM! It charged right away!*

Your exploration

Of course, it is not a given that you will be affected by an acute illness while you are immersing yourself in this book or getting to grips with your heart rate variability data. If, however, one day you should notice that something is brewing, go ahead and get this book out again and re-read this chapter. If you are clearly sick, see if you can discern a change in your heart rate variability or stress level. Many patients with monitors have told me how the readings on the watch reacted before they themselves noticed any symptoms. Then keep an eye on how long it takes before the data is all the way back to where it was before the outbreak of the illness. This way you can learn more about how your body responds to illness. If your health was already poor to begin with, it may take you longer to recover.

Try different strategies to relieve the work your body does while you are ill. Sleep longer than you usually do. What happens when you add in a few power naps? Or how about some breathing exercises? Eat lighter meals and avoid alcohol. Before you return to exercising again, start slowly with a leisurely walk – preferably one you already have some data on so you can make a comparison. Make a game out of finding out how you can assist your body to get better. And if you have to go to the doctor, feel free to show the results you have had so that the two of you can work together on mapping out your further plans for either working or going on sick leave.

A monitor can endow you with more power as a patient and at the same time a greater responsibility for your own recovery. My distinct impression is that those who truly take on this responsibility are also the healthiest people. Try to take this as encouragement to take control!

Bente (48)
I have fibromyalgia and I am 50% disabled. During the first round of collecting data, I took the smallest possible dose of Sarotex (50 mg). My Body Battery was rarely over 40, as a rule it was usually under 25. Regardless of what I did, the Body Battery was often empty for three days. Then I quit taking Sarotex and there was a clear increase in the Body Battery. Now I am able to get up to 70 or 80.*

*NB If you find HRV results that indicate that your medication dosage may need altering, please consult your doctor before making any changes.

STAGE EIGHT: WEIGHT CONTROL

At my practice, I unfortunately meet a significant over-representation of overweight people. This is probably related to the fact that they are ill more often than other people, and perhaps because an incredible 70% of us are carrying around too much weight at the moment. Over the nearly 25 years that I have worked as a doctor, this development has been formidable to see. Whereas previously weeks went by between each time I saw an alarmingly overweight patient at my practice, it has now become a daily occurrence. The severity of this epidemic has probably not even begun to manifest itself fully. For example, it took 40 to 50 years of widespread cigarette use before the full extent of smoking's adverse consequences came to light.

The science
There are two types of adipose tissue. One is called subcutaneous fat. This lies under the skin, and it is relatively harmless. The second one, which is much more harmful, is mostly located in the belly and is called visceral fat. This kind of fat settles around the body's organs. It is especially dangerous if it is deposited in the liver.

Incidences of fatty liver used to occur due to alcohol abuse. Now we increasingly see fatty livers in younger people including children, without alcohol consumption being in the picture. The cause for this is the consumption of fast-release carbohydrates which increase the level of insulin in the blood and subsequently stimulate the liver to store fat.

While subcutaneous fat consists of a fairly passive storage of fatty acids, visceral fat secretes inflammatory substances that are carried around the body in the blood. These inflammatory substances are secreted because each fat cell stores more fat than it was made to hold. The cell's mitochondria become overloaded and send inflammatory signals out as if the cell was ill. Fatty substances also leak from the cells into the bloodstream. The fat sticks to the blood vessel walls, which then narrow. This increases the risk of disease and results in poorer heart rate variability.

From the doctor's practice

My experience at my practice tells me that, while diets do not work, losing weight as a consequence of making lasting changes in one's lifestyle does produce good results. However, we cannot quite escape the need to keep an eye on our body weight; managing to keep the new weight stable requires daily effort. I have found that either we strive a little every day to maintain our normal weight or we will struggle heavily every day by carrying too much weight. The latter alternative creates the most dissatisfaction and disease over time. Weight loss requires a long-term effort which can save you from dying prematurely. Data has shown that heart rate variability improves in step with weight loss.

My exploration

Apart from fasting, weighing myself every day is my most important tactic for losing weight. By doing this I am instantly able to perceive any weight gain. If I do gain weight, I will fast for half a day and then my weight is back to its normal level. This strategy was of great help to me when I was trying to lose 20 kilos. When I recall accomplishing this, I remember feeling excited about not having to carry around the weight equivalent of a whole item of checked-in luggage every time I took a step! It took me over two years to do this and maintaining it still requires daily effort. But just the pleasure of seeing my chest stick out in front of my stomach is reward enough for me.

My scales also measure my body fat percentage. I have a Tanita scale, after testing several others that were not as precise (among the more affordable brands, Beurer is also good). Through sending a small amount of electricity through my body via a handle, the Tanita scale estimates the amount of water, muscle, and fat in my body and then calculates my biological age. For example, it showed me that the 4 kilos I lost during two months in which I did not exercise consisted only of muscle mass. Tanita also makes a small travel scale that is useful for me since I travel so often. Consequently, this summer for the first time I was able to maintain my weight during a three-week holiday. When I weigh myself as part of my morning routine it takes just 30 seconds – and in doing so I have made a big effort for the sake of my health.

I found that the biggest problem I face is dealing with temptation in the days in between and around the holidays, when I am outside my usual routine. This is consistent with what research has discovered. A typical American puts on two-thirds of all the weight he or she gains in a year in the period between Thanksgiving and New Year's Eve, even though this period makes up no more than one-sixth of the year. In the same way, I could easily gain 4 or 5 kilos during the Christmas holidays. It has become a lot easier for me to enter the New Year in balance since I began to slot in some fasting days in between the ones where we are gathered together during Christmas break. Every day I cut out drinkable calories and I prefer a low-carbohydrate diet. For lunch I would rather eat a salad and some nuts as a snack between meals.

Your exploration

Go out and get yourself a modern scale that measures body fat percentage and muscle mass. Studies show that people lose an average of 6 to 7 kilos just by weighing themselves daily. All this stepping on a scale keeps the desire to lose weight firmly in the front of our frontal lobes so that we are better able to resist chocolate and sweets and choose to eat an apple instead. As I have said before – what you can measure, you can master! I do not think it is a coincidence that most of the obese patients I meet at my practice have no idea how much they weigh – and they are often shocked when they find out what their weight actually is – while people of normal weight tend to maintain a good overview of it. However, obesity is such a delicate subject, as well as being one loaded with shame, that I and most other doctors avoid broaching it during consultations. I choose to point it out here because it affects our state of health so strongly and because we can measure the effects of weight loss with a heart rate variability monitor.

Here is a tip for those of you who use food to regulate high stress levels, or if you are a comfort eater. When you feel the need to eat because you are stressed out or because you feel sad or upset, first try to do some breathing exercises to calm your nerves. Afterwards you can see if your desire to eat is still there.

How to test whether the fat you have is mostly subcutaneous fat or dangerous visceral fat

1. Grab your belly fat. If it feels like a pillow when you squeeze it in your hand, then it is mostly subcutaneous fat. If it is more like squeezing a hard ball, then you probably have more visceral fat.
2. A more exact way to find out is to ask your GP to measure the ratio between triglycerides and HDL-cholesterol in your blood. If you have a bad case of obesity, this ratio will be over two. The closer you are to one, and preferably under it, the better it is for you.

STAGE NINE: NICOTINE

Cigarette smoking in Norway exploded in the 1930s and reached its peak in the 1960s when 60% of men and 40% of women smoked. People paying money to fill their delicate lungs, which contain 500 million microscopic air sacs, with poisonous smoke full of tar is almost too incredible to be true. Right now, less than 10% of Norway's population smoke and only 1–2% of young people between the ages of 16 and 24 do. However, 15% of Norwegian people between 16 and 74 use snus, a smokeless wet powder that you place under your top lip. In the UK, vaping is more popular, with 9.1% of adults (equivalent to 4.7 million people) using e-cigarettes in 2023, the highest rate ever.

How does nicotine affect us? What impact does it have on our health? How can it affect our stress level? We are going to look at some common secondary diseases caused by tobacco use, but we will place particular emphasis on examining how smoking, snus, and tobacco substitutes like sprays, vapes, and chewing gum impact our daily body budget.

And do we in fact become calmer through having a cigarette or a vape? Follow along and you will get an answer or two to these questions.

Tore (35)
I use snus and for quite some time I have had my suspicions that doing so may exacerbate the stress I have. I have now tried going cold turkey and after a few days of withdrawal it looks like my stress level and heart rate are lower than they were before. I also feel that I am sleeping better and have a more even level of energy throughout the day.

The science

A daily smoker shortens his or her life by up to 10 years. Each cigarette that is smoked for 6 minutes can shorten one's life by 15 minutes, i.e. a 70-year-old who has smoked for 50 years may have spent 4 years of his or her life to make it 10 years shorter. On top of the health costs of smoking comes all the money spent on tobacco products.

Nicotine affects the autonomic nervous system so that it releases the adrenaline and dopamine hormones, both of which give us a euphoric and addictive kick. Nicotine causes the musculature in the blood vessel walls to contract. Blood flow is decreased and the blood pressure in the arteries (the blood vessels going from the heart and out to the body) increases. The result of this is high blood pressure and an increased heart rate. In nature, nicotine is in fact a poison that plants use as an insecticide.

For many years the tobacco industry managed to manipulate medical science into believing that smoking was good for people's health. Since the serious harmful effects of smoking only become apparent after several decades of using it, it took time before people realised how effectively smoking could decrease their life expectancy. So far, 70 different substances have been found in tobacco smoke that can cause serious disease. In total, more than 7,000 different chemicals have been identified in a cigarette.

Tobacco smoke physically destroys the lungs, which are clearly the most vulnerable part of our body where tiny alveoli take in oxygen and distribute it to the blood. The nicotine causes arteriosclerosis in which the blood vessels constrict so that the supply of blood to the body's organs, including the skin, worsens. For example, it takes much longer for wounds to heal after an operation if you smoke, and the risk of infection also increases. It is widely known that smoking causes and predisposes a person to Chronic Obstructive Pulmonary Disease (COPD), heart disease, lung cancer, and arteriosclerosis. Smoking and nicotine also increase insulin resistance and contribute to increased inflammation in the body.

Since 2004, when a total ban on smoking in bars and restaurants in Norway went into effect, most nicotine addicts have fortunately switched to using snus. Snus is considered to have only 10% of the potential to damage one's health that cigarettes have. Nevertheless, it appears that using snus puts stress on the autonomic nervous system, which in turn can lead to a number of the inflammatory-related diseases that I have mentioned so often in this book. The question is, of course, whether using snus is harmful for you. And this is something that a heart rate monitor can show you. The degree to which using snus causes stress and reduces one's willpower is dependent on the individual. For me, using snus reduced my disposable energy considerably – and it felt pointless to waste my valuable energy processing the stress resulting from using snus instead of it being spent on more useful tasks.

You might think that the average life expectancy would have shot up now that nearly everyone has stopped smoking, but the other lifestyle diseases seem to have tempered this increase. The sofa, the screen, diet, and loneliness all seem to be as toxic as a pack of cigarettes.

From the doctor's practice

There is rarely a reason to ask a patient if they smoke; the answer can be found in his or her face. A smoker in their 50s or 60s often looks 10 years older than a non-smoker of the same age. In this respect, a person's external appearance reflects what is going on internally due to smoking cutting off the supply of blood to both the skin and the body's delicate machinery, thus contributing to the presence of more wrinkles, less elasticity in the skin, and a situation in which inner organs, unfortunately, are just as prune-like in appearance as the skin of a smoker.

Smokers have often argued that smoking relieves stress. But smoking relieves nothing more than a craving for nicotine because people who use tobacco products often seem to me to be more stressed than other people. And that's not so strange when you think about it, because their lives are on a nicotine-fuelled roller-coaster ride. For them, the stress is double. When they have not had a dose of nicotine, they become mentally stressed due to withdrawal. And when they finally do get some, their nervous system is activated, thus stressing the body.

> **Henrikke (38)**
> I stopped using snus in the middle of April and saw my daily resting heart rate drop from 70 to 60.

My exploration

On a normally windy day during my residency in Bodø, I sought shelter in the Glasshuset, which is an indoor, glass-covered shopping arcade. I checked my pockets: a pack of Lucky Strikes, a container of snus, a nicotine patch for my upper arm, nicotine gum . . . and I had just that minute bought a nicotine nasal spray at the chemist's in a desperate attempt to quit smoking. This was the first time I'd tried nicotine spray, and I regretted it immediately. It was like putting pepper spray up my nose. My eyes watered, and then I pulled myself together and tried to find the quickest way out of there.

For years my countless attempts to quit smoking were futile. Every time I tried to stop using nicotine, I would become depressed and not feel like myself. During my residency, I switched to using snus daily since there were so few opportunities to have a cigarette break. Maybe I needed the kick from the nicotine to keep my attention up through the hectic 24-hour shifts. In 2004 when I went on a pilgrimage to Santiago, I packed ten containers of snus in my rucksack. When I ran out near the end, I had to resort to Lucky Strikes again. Even while I was walking, I smoked 40 cigarettes a day.

Over the years, and especially after I had children, it became obvious that being a slave to nicotine cost me far too much in the way of time, money, and energy. I wanted to decide for myself what I wanted to do; I did not want my choices ruled by an idiotic molecule of nicotine!

Since then I have cracked and given in only occasionally, and only when I was working at an emergency unit far from home and out of my wife's sight. But eventually it struck me that the shifts where I used snus were the most tiring ones and that it was the snus – and not the burden of dealing with patients – that was the common denominator among them. Using my heart rate monitor I discovered that on the days I used snus it was nearly impossible to read and differentiate between the other stresses. The effect of the nicotine activated my nervous system so powerfully that it was running on high gear and neither breathing exercises nor power naps were able to mute its effect. The impact of this lasted long into the night, disturbed my sleep, and contributed to me not being fully recovered when I woke up. However, since I wanted to investigate the effect of various stresses on the nervous system, it was only natural to pop into the shop and get a pack of cigarettes – all in the name of scientific research, you understand!

After being shocked by how much more expensive cigarettes had become since I last bought them, I had another shock in store. It did not take too many drags before I got an answer as to whether nicotine had an activating or calming effect on my nervous system. The stress activation on my monitor went right through the roof, and it was not until a few hours later that I was back in a resting state. The next two cigarettes produced the same effect, only somewhat weaker. If I had started smoking regularly again, then my body would have become accustomed to the stress and the results of doing it would have probably evened themselves out more. But even for science I am not willing to test this to find out if this would be the case.

Your exploration

Now, of course, I am not going to encourage you to try tobacco. Nicotine has been shown to be just as addictive as heroin. No other poisonous substance is ingested as regularly by its users. If you already smoke, vape, or use snus, however, try going a week without nicotine and notice how this affects your nervous system. Bear in mind that your heart rate monitor may not show any relevant data until the end of the week, since the first few days are likely to be affected by withdrawal. Notice to what extent cutting out nicotine affects your sleep, your willpower, and how tired you feel. Here is a tip for those of you who think it is difficult to stay away from it: when the nicotine craving appears, wait ten minutes, and see if the craving is still just as strong. Try to distract yourself from the craving by doing something else, such as ten squats or breathing exercises for two minutes.

If you use up 10 minutes on smoking a cigarette, including the time it may take to find one and then move to a place where you can smoke, and smoke 10 of them a day, your smoking-related activities will in total amount to 100 minutes a day, 700 minutes a week, and 36,500 minutes a year. In 10 years, that will amount to 365,000 minutes, or in other words 6,000 hours, almost 36 weeks you could have used on something a lot more sensible. (And on top of that, statistically you will have shaved 15,000 hours (one and a half years) from your lifespan for every decade you smoke. Six smoking decades would steal 9 years from your lifetime. And if you smoke 20 a day, according to a Dutch study, you risk cutting 13 years from your lifetime.) What could you have achieved otherwise with 6,000 hours of effort at your disposal? Created a masterpiece? Made your dream come true? It may be helpful for you to keep this thought in mind when you are attacked by a nicotine craving and have to choose whether or not to light up another cigarette. This small, seemingly innocent choice, repeated over the years, can make the difference between achieving what you want to do in life or not doing it at all. For you, a big carrot on the stick is this: the human body is extremely good at cleaning up the mess you have made in your lungs and the rest of your body, and that 7 years after having your last cigarette, the risk of dying prematurely is just the same as if you had never smoked at all. So, the longer you have smoked, the more years of your life you can save by quitting. For example, if you are 55 years old and have smoked for 35 years, there is a great risk that you only have 15 years left to live. If you quit, chances are good that you will still have 30 years left. That is twice as many!

At least, that is what I find solace in.

Here is another way I can support myself to not start up again based on my experience at my practice: the patients who do not quit smoking, even after suffering a heart attack, will have their next heart attack long before the ones who have managed to quit. Often, the difference between the two is ten years. Many of them are even able to rid themselves of heart disease completely and consequently never suffer another heart attack at all.

When it comes to vaping and snus, we have far less reliable figures to look at. But if you are like me, you will be struck by the fact that each day that you live nicotine-free is one in which you have more energy at your disposal than you did before.

Recommended reading
Allen Carr's Easy Way to Stop Smoking by Allen Carr

Some predetermined factors

AGEING

At the start of this book, I touched upon the difference between biological and chronological ageing. Even though we can slow down the speed at which ageing proceeds, and even turn our biological clock back in some areas, it is obviously not possible to stop time or the days from passing. So, I will take as my starting point the idea that you are now doing what you can with regard to your biological age and concentrate on ageing, which is something humans are unable to influence.

In the table overleaf, you can study the average heart rate variability of men and women at various ages. The statistical expression *standard deviation* means, for example, that a woman between the ages of 35 and 44 will have an average of 35.4 milliseconds (ms), but that it is within the normal range to be between 16.9 and 53.9 ms (standard deviation is ±18,5). RMSSD is the most widely used measurement for heart rate variability.

The HRV value decreases steadily with age. This is a sign that, as we age, our sympathetic activation gradually increases and the physiology has to work harder and harder to obtain a balance in the body account. Perhaps this is due to the body having to expend more and more energy on maintenance and repair, for which we needed less energy in our youth. Our cells have to work harder to maintain the same functioning. Yet, although we need more time for recovery after exerting ourselves than we did in our younger days, we still require a certain amount of movement and sufficient stress to be able to avoid declining physically and mentally.

While lifestyle diseases at a young age are often induced and maintained by living at a high tempo and stress level, it tends to be the opposite in old age, in which passivity and too little stress create illnesses. Many people age much faster than is necessary.

In old age, it will be difficult to get our heart rate variability to be on the same level it was when we were younger. However, an older person who exercises regularly and works to have a good stress balance may be capable of having their heart rate variability be just as good as the one the much younger, stressed, sleepless, and out-of-shape version of themselves had.

Normal values in the population			
Age	Gender	RMSSD (ms)	Standard deviation (ms)
25–34	Men	39.7	± 19.9
	Women	42.9	± 22.8
35–44	Men	32	± 16.5
	Women	35.4	± 18.5
45–54	Men	23	± 10.9
	Women	26.3	± 13.6
55–64	Men	19.9	± 11.1
	Women	21.4	± 11.9
65–74	Men	19.1	± 10.7
	Women	19.1	± 11.8

Source: Voss, Schroeder, Heitmann, Peters and Perz: Voss norm study of gender and age, 2015

> **Eva (60)**
> I'm about to make a big statement. Looking at data and having a focus has changed my life. The change from running around as much as possible to resting as soon as I am able to is something I have experienced as being very positive. Knowing that living through stressful and demanding periods in my life is OK as long as I follow them up with sufficient recovery is also a change that benefits my body. This is something I am 100% convinced about.

Biological age

Chronological ageing is a process over which we have no control. Time passes, regardless of our trying to interfere with it. On the other hand, it is possible to influence biological ageing. Many of the diseases that are caused by premature ageing are ones that would possibly have appeared at a certain point in time, but if you look after your biological age then maybe you will contract them between the ages of 70 and 90 instead of 50. A good, solid, and supportive physiology will not just increase the likelihood of you living longer, you may also have more healthy years to live thrown into the bargain. People are wrong when they claim that any extra years they get will be spent in a nursing home and are therefore not really worth putting in the effort for.

Inflammaging is a much-used term in popular medical literature. It indicates that much of the cause of what we call ageing is due to diseases that are caused by inflammatory reactions in the body, which can actually be avoided. In other words, what is going on is that inflammation-triggered diseases are being misinterpreted as ageing. This is what I see through my own personal observation at my practice and when I hold photography courses: 75-year-old patients or photography course participants who move like someone who is 25, and the opposite, 25-year-old people who climb up stairs as if they were 75. This is rarely due to a coincidence. It is often one's lifestyle that dictates who is going to end up in which of these two categories.

If your biological clock can remain below your biological age for decades, then there is a good chance you will have a long, healthy life, perhaps with the exception of the last two or three years. And several heart rate monitors can give you an estimate of your biological age based on your fitness scores.

As an A&E emergency physician, I often have to write death certificates. Meeting relatives of the deceased who managed to live past the age of 90 triggers my curiosity. Many of those I have spoken to have told me that their loved one was able to live on their own at home until their very last years alive. As a rule, these elderly people had plenty of exercise through doing natural activities such as physical work and going on walks, they had hobbies and a rich social life, were always smiling, they ate healthily and prudently, got sufficient sleep, and had a winning personality with an aura that radiated that they were at peace with themselves. Often, the sons and daughters of the deceased sat on the sofa and expressed their joy over having inherited such good genes. However, a quick investigation into this reveals a different truth: depending on their lifestyle choices they may be up to 20 biological years older than their chronological age suggests. Studies have shown that only 3% of the variation of a person's lifespan can be attributed to their parents' genes. Even among twins we are able to find a 15-year variation in lifespan. Lifestyle is the determining factor in this area.

People's attitude towards becoming older is an important factor in ageing. Research has shown that the people who have a positive attitude towards old age tend to live seven years longer than those who have a negative attitude towards it (this is corrected for state of health, depression, socioeconomic status, and other possible factors). This is likely connected to the fact that people who have a positive view on getting older and associate words like 'wise' and 'capable' to elderly people more easily exercise and follow the advice of their doctor. People who associate ageing with words such as 'useless' and 'closed-minded' will to a lesser degree believe that they can play an active role in the development of their health.

A research project looked at what impact these two extremes of attitude may have during an acute health crisis, such as a hip fracture, lung disease, or cancer. Patients who had a positive view of ageing responded to a situation such as this by increasing their efforts to look after their health. And the opposite of this was true – negatively predisposed patients were even less motivated to make an effort. In a way, a person could somehow manage to 'think' their way into improving their health since these thoughts do lead to actions that promote healing.

SEASONAL VARIATION

Something I have discovered through my own data is that my heart rate variability is better in the summer. Oura, WHOOP, and Garmin can all confirm my findings. Is the variability due to people being more exposed to disease in the winter? We in the healthcare system have long emphasised that, as people stay indoors more during the winter, there is a greater likelihood for them to infect each other. In addition, the flu thrives particularly well during that season.

The number of deaths in the winter is significantly higher than in the summer. It has been assumed that this is due to influenza. However, could it also be the case that a general reduction in physiological and immunological capacity plays a part in this, and that this makes us more vulnerable to a number of diseases? Could the increased levels of inflammatory-inducing cytokines that have been measured in the blood of Europeans also be a contributing factor? What if this increased level of inflammation was due to the advanced mobilisation of the immune system prior to an expected higher level of infection pressure?

Hopefully, we will soon be able to get some significant answers to these questions now that millions of people who live in a similar part of the world use heart rate monitors.

The reason why HRV values are higher in the summer is equally unclear. In fact, it turns out that we sleep less during this time of year and yet recover better. We apparently need less sleep to maintain the same heart rate variability. Perhaps it is the amount of sunlight that is affecting us, or the D vitamins that are made in our skin? Going shirtless in the sun has also been shown to increase our sex hormones. Half of the sun's light consists of infrared light, which has been found to improve the functioning of mitochondria (the cells' power station). Perhaps we can do something to even out the seasonal differences, but for now what is most important is to be aware that, in general, we will be somewhat weaker in the winter, and we need to take that into account. In that part of the year, we need a little more sleep and can tolerate stress a little less. For that reason, it does not appear particularly smart to choose a low point such as January as the time to change your lifestyle after making an optimistic New Year's resolution. After all, that is when we have the least energy, and our willpower is at its weakest. What if we instead formulated what we wished to accomplish sitting in front of the fireplace in January, made plans for actualising it in March and then began working on it in May? Following this, we could have a greater chance to succeed.

GENDER

Men consistently have a lower heart rate variability than women – at least until the difference is evened out by age. As we can see in the table above, 'Voss norm study of gender and age' from 2015, women's heart rate variability is 3–3.5 milliseconds above the men's all the way up to menopause. This may be a factor that contributes to men dying on average two to three years before women do. Perhaps this explains why men have a more aggressive immune system, more cytokines in their blood and more inflammation in their bodies. Historically, this has been the case because men were more often susceptible to becoming injured while hunting or going to war and were more likely to engage in risk-taking behaviour which could lead to them becoming injured and contracting injury-related infections. Men thus needed a more 'flammable' immune system. This defence system often tends to 'shoot at anything that moves', and in the process inadvertently damages innocent tissue.

Through evolution, women to a greater extent have been vulnerable to disease that sneaks up on them slowly. Therefore, their immune systems do not need to react quite as quickly. Biologically, it has also been more important for the tribe's survival that women live the longest. The men's task has largely been completed once they have ensured that they have impregnated a woman.

Evolutionary biologists in fact think women's menopause is a consequence of grandmothers having time to take care of their grandchildren and thereby strengthening the prospects of the entire tribe's survival. This trait then evolved in the human genome.

Humans are the only land mammals who go through menopause. The other species that do are whales. And among them grandmothers occupy a central role as childminders too.

> **Bente (48)**
> I found that hot flushes from menopause turn out to cause stress and empty the Body Battery.

MENSTRUATION

While menstruation is a subject that might be considered to be limited to female readers of childbearing age, it nevertheless concerns us all. I have seen how strongly these monthly bleedings can reduce the capacity of many girls and women during busy and vulnerable periods in their lives.

One explanation as to why researchers who develop medications have largely used men as guinea pigs is that their research findings could easily have become distorted by the significant physiological variations women experience during their menstrual cycle. These variations also show up loud and clear on our heart rate monitors: bodily preparations for a possible pregnancy do not in fact take place in quiet isolation. The body puts in a powerful effort.

In the first half of the menstrual cycle, a woman's heart rate variability will be more like that of a man's. This phase is often called the *low hormone phase*, or the *follicular phase*, and is characterised by its relaxed state, parasympathetic activation, and its attendant higher heart rate variability. In the second half, after ovulation, the *high hormone phase*, or *luteal phase*, begins. This phase is distinguished by the activation of the sympathetic nervous system. Preparations are made in the body for a pregnancy shortly after this. The heart rate variability may drop, and the body budget becomes depleted. In this part of the menstrual cycle, it may be a good idea to take it easy.

Note that if you use hormonal contraceptives, ovulation will stop, and the stressful luteal phase will end. The hormones in the contraceptives will still be able to affect your mood. This is a common side effect.

The menstrual problems which are most often brought up at the doctor's practice are the tendency to suffer from migraines and general fatigue. Students often say that they struggle to find the energy to do their schoolwork, especially the week before bleeding occurs.

The menstrual cycle is thus not just a matter of mood swings but something that affects disposable energy that may be used for any purpose. And in general, too little attention has been directed towards adapting one's level of activity according to available energy.

You might want to keep an eye on whether there is any pattern in your heart rate variability that repeats during your menstrual cycle. It may be interesting in particular to compare the weeks before and after the bleeding starts. If you use birth control pills, then your menstruation is artificially induced due to the hormones having tricked your body into believing it is pregnant – but without the body getting to complete its preparatory work for a pregnancy. According to WHOOP's data, women using birth control pills have a heart rate variability curve that is more like the curve of a man.

If you have a chronic disease that comes in waves, such as, for example, migraines, fibromyalgia, irritable bowel syndrome, or depression, it may be useful to observe the link between heart rate variability, menstruation, and your symptoms.

You should avoid exercising strenuously in the last week before your period when your HRV may be low. In fact, the HRV numbers show, contrary to what one might think, that recovery is optimal during the time of bleeding. But if you think about it carefully, the following makes sense: the body has finished its task, a pregnancy did not take place and now it can sit back and relax, at least for a couple of weeks, until its next hopeful attempt. In the period leading up to the next luteal phase, energies can more easily be allocated for exercising or other stresses.

As more and more women use heart rate monitors and work out, we will certainly get more answers as to how menstruation affects surplus energy which can be utilised for exercise and other physiological stresses.

10 great tips for excellent health

1. Make sure you get eight hours of sound sleep. Ideally, go to bed by 10.00 p.m.
2. Dim the lights and wind down the intensity of your activities after 8.00 p.m.
3. Limit your eating window to eight hours, such as between 11.00 a.m. and 7.00 p.m.
4. Do some strength training every day.
5. Walk at a brisk pace for half an hour three times a week.
6. Make room for 15 minutes of relaxing activities a day.
7. Eat a varied plant-based diet. Avoid ultra-processed foods.
8. Finish your shower with two to three minutes of exposure to ice-cold water.
9. Only drink alcohol on special occasions.
10. Visit natural surroundings for half an hour a day, preferably during the daytime.

Your ten changes

1. _____

2. _____

3. _____

4. _____

5. _____

6. _____

7. _____

8. _____

9. _____

10. _____

thepulsecure.com

You do not have to let your expedition end here! Throughout this entire book you have read what the people in the test group have discovered about their physiology. They have shared their findings in a Facebook group as well as learning from each other and from webinars I have held. This has been such a success that I have created a website where this work will continue. There, you can make a profile, post questions, share photos of your heart rate variability curves and get input from others. Online courses and webinars will be given where you can learn more about how you can use a monitor to forge your way to better health.

Unfortunately, there are all too many people who struggle with getting their physiology in balance for any healthcare system to be able to solve this issue alone. If we can learn from each other, the process will move forward much more quickly. You are most welcome to meet the other members of this expedition at www.thepulsecure.com!

Therese (42)
The best thing about monitoring my heart rate variability is the feeling that it is like having a hearing aid attached to my body. And now that I can hear my body's signals, I am much better able to take care of myself!

The way forward – strength to follow your dreams!

You have now gained insight into how you can use artificial intelligence to improve your health. In the years ahead, these tools will increase in number and be improved upon. Just as computers have managed to make both flight and air traffic control safer, artificial intelligence will also help us improve our health much more than the healthcare system is able to do today. Hopefully, it will prevent so many diseases that your doctor will be able to use more of his or her time being a consultant and life coach for you as you take control of your own health.

I hope that through using this book and heart rate monitors you have established a better balance of energy and are able to notice the presence of an increased surplus of energy in your everyday life, and that you are able to use your energy for something more than just keeping your head above the water. In the grand scheme of things, our time on Earth is relatively short, so you and I should try to live as adventurous a life as possible. After all, we are living in conditions and have opportunities that the previous 12,000 generations of people before us could not even come close to.

So, what do you want to use your surplus energy on? What dreams do you want to see come true? Maybe some of them are big, expensive, and time-consuming? Can you come up with a plan to make them a reality? A goal without a plan tends to remain just a dream. Do you have a small dream that you can make happen today? Something you can see, hear, or experience right now? Magic is all around us, always – all we have to do is open our eyes and see it!

As knowledge becomes more widespread and accessible throughout society, the difference between those who know a lot about health and those who know only a little will unfortunately increase. I can already see a strong tendency towards this development at my practice. The health-conscious people are fitter and healthier than ever while those who neglect their health and have little interest in gaining knowledge of this type are weaker and sicker. Feel free to spread knowledge to your family and friends about how they can gain increased well-being and a capacity to carry things out through an awareness of how to manage stress and use heart rate monitors. Inspire them to set out on the same journey you have chosen. And if you have the opportunity to embark on an adventure, take someone with you!

Finally, I would like to thank you for completing the stages in this book. You have now passed the physiological driving test. But even if you are now better equipped than before to navigate an at times chaotic physiological universe, a long time yet remains before you will be a truly experienced driver of your physiology. Be patient – there is no road to mastery other than the one where you collect a few small dings and scratches as well as survive some pretty big collisions along the way. Do not let disappointment stop you. That is what you will learn from the most.

I wish you the best of luck!

Thanks

A special thanks to my immediate family, who have had to put up with me looking more like a robot than a human being, with up to eight measuring instruments on my body at the same time.

Thanks to my other family, friends and acquaintances who have tolerated me asking about the state of their Body Battery before I even asked how they were doing.

Many thanks to all the 198 'test pilots' who contributed with their anecdotes, and provided feedback on the drafts of this book along the way.

Thanks also to Audun Myskja, Sigrun Haaland, Anne Spurkland, Inge Lindseth, Annette Dragland, Jarle Holt, Lise Galaasen and Øivind Arneberg.

Recommended podcasts

Feel Better, Live More
The Diary of a CEO
The Doctor's Kitchen Podcast
The Doctor's Farmacy
Huberman Lab
The Peter Attia Drive
The Resetter Podcast
The Rich Roll Podcast
WHOOP Podcast

If you search my name on your podcast app, you will quickly be able to find the podcasts on which I appear as a guest. Most of them will of course be in Norwegian, but a growing number will be in English.

You can also follow me here:
Instagram: @the_pulse_cure
Facebook: dr.torkil
www. thepulsecure.com

Bibliography

The brain and the nervous system

Bullmore, Edward: *The Inflamed Mind: A Radical New Approach to Depression.* Short Books 2019

Kamath, Markad, et al.: *Heart Rate Variability Signal Analysis: Clinical Applications.* CRC Press 2012

Mayer, Emeran: *The Mind-Gut Connection: How the Hidden Conversation Within Our Bodies Impacts Our Mood, Our Choices, and Our Overall Health.* Harper Wave 2018

Palmer, Christopher: *Brain Energy: A Revolutionary Breakthrough in Understanding Mental Health—and Improving Treatment for Anxiety, Depression, OCD, PTSD, and More.* BenBella Books 2022

Sapolsky, Robert: *Behave: The Biology of Humans at Our Best and Worst.* Vintage 2018

Sapolsky, Robert: *Why Zebras Don't Get Ulcers.* St. Martin's Press 2004

The immune system

Macciochi, Jenna: *Immunity: The Science of Staying Well.* HarperNonFiction 2020

Macciochi, Jenna: *Your Blueprint for Strong Immunity: Personalise Your Diet and Lifestyle for Better Health.* Yellow Kite 2022

Mayer, Emeran: *The Gut-Immune Connection: How Understanding the Connection Between Food and Immunity Can Help Us Regain Our Health.* Harper 2021

Evolutionary perspective

Breuning, Loretta Graziano: *I, Mammal: How to Make Peace with the Animal Urge for Social Power*. Inner Mammal Institute 2011

Godfrey-Smith, Peter: *Metazoa: Animal Minds and the Birth of Consciousness*. William Collins 2021

Hansen, Anders: *The Happiness Cure: Why You're Not Built for Constant Happiness, and How to Find a Way Through*. Vermilion 2023

Ilardi, Steve: *The Depression Cure: The Six-Step Programme to Beat Depression without Drugs*. Vermilion 2010

Natterson-Horowitz, Barbara and Bowers, Kathryn: *Zoobiquity: The Astonishing Connection Between Animal and Human Health*. Vintage 2013

Nesse, Randolph M.: *Good Reasons for Bad Feelings: Insights from the Frontier of Evolutionary Psychiatry*. Penguin Books 2020

Riddle, Tony: *Be More Human: How to Transform Your Lifestyle for Optimum Health, Happiness and Vitality*. Penguin Life 2022

Von Hippel, William: *The Social Leap: The New Evolutionary Science of Who We Are, Where We Come From, and What Makes Us Happy*. HarperWave 2018

Psychology

Barrett, Lisa Feldman: *How Emotions Are Made: The Secret Life of the Brain*. Pan Books 2018

Barrett, Lisa Feldman: *Seven and a Half Lessons About the Brain*. Picador 2021

Breuning, Loretta: *Tame Your Anxiety: Rewiring Your Brain for Happiness*. Rowman & Littlefield 2019

Hari, Johann: *Lost Connections: Uncovering the Real Causes of Depression – and the Unexpected Solutions*. Bloomsbury Circus 2018

Joseph, Stephen: *What Doesn't Kill Us: A Guide to Overcoming Adversity and Moving Forward*. Piatkus 2013

Kashdan, Todd: *The Upside of Your Dark Side: Why Being Your Whole Self – Not Just Your "Good" Self – Drives Success and Fulfillment*. Plume Books 2015

Van der Kolk, Bessel: *The Body Keeps the Score: Mind, Brain and Body in the Healing of Trauma*. Penguin Books 2015

Seligman, Martin: *Flourish: A New Understanding of Happiness and Well-Being – and How To Achieve Them*. Nicholas Brealey Publishing 2011

Seligman, Martin: *Learned Optimism: How to Change Your Mind and Your Life*. Nicholas Brealey Publishing 2018

Siegel, Daniel J.: *Mindsight: The New Science of Personal Transformation*. Bantam Books 2010

General health

Attia, Peter: *Outlive: The Science and Art of Longevity*. Vermilion 2023

Blackburn, Elizabeth: *The Telomere Effect: A Revolutionary Approach to Living Younger, Healthier, Longer*. Orion Spring 2018

Bryson, Bill: *The Body: A Guide for Occupants*. Doubleday 2019

Enders, Giulia: *Gut: The Inside Story of Our Body's Most Under-rated Organ*. Scribe UK 2016

Furman, Richard: *Prescription for Life: Three Simple Strategies to Live Younger Longer*. Revell 2015

Gottfried, Sara: *The Hormone Cure*. Scribner 2014

Rediger, Jeff: *Cured: The Power of Our Immune System and the Mind-Body Connection*. Penguin Life 2021

Critical perspective on the healthcare system

Abramson, John: *Sickening: How Big Pharma Broke American Health Care and How We Can Repair It*. Mariner Books 2022

Wootton, David: *Bad Medicine: Doctors Doing Harm Since Hippocrates*. Oxford University Press 2007

Life skills

Baumeister, Roy and Tierney, John: *Willpower: Rediscovering Our Greatest Strength*. Allen Lane 2012

Brown, Brené: *The Gifts of Imperfection: Let Go of Who You Think You're Supposed to Be and Embrace Who You Are*. Vermilion 2020

Brown, Stuart: *Play: How It Shapes the Brain, Opens the Imagination, and Invigorates the Soul.* Penguin Publishing Group 2010

Buettner, Dan: *Thrive: Finding Happiness the Blue Zones Way.* National Geographic Society 2011

Cain, Susan: *Quiet: The Power of Introverts in a World That Can't Stop Talking.* Crown 2012

Canfield, Jack: *The Success Principles: How to Get from Where You Are to Where You Want to Be.* HarperNonFiction 2005

Carnegie, Dale: *How to Stop Worrying and Start Living.* Ebury Publishing 2004

Carnegie, Dale: *How to Win Friends and Influence People.* Penguin Books 2004

Dispenza, Joe: *Breaking the Habit of Being Yourself: How to Lose Your Mind and Create a New One.* Hay House 2013

Dispenza, Joe: *You Are the Placebo: Making Your Mind Matter.* Hay House 2014

Duckworth, Angela: *Grit: The Power of Passion and Perseverance.* Scribner 2016

Dweck, Carol S.: *Mindset: Changing the Way You Think to Fulfil Your Potential.* Robinson 2017

Dyer, Wayne: *Excuses Begone!: How to Change Lifelong, Self-Defeating Thinking Habits.* Hay House 2009

Garcia, Hector: *Ikigai: The Japanese Secret to a Long and Happy Life.* Hutchinson 2017

Gray, Peter: *Free to Learn: Why Unleashing the Instinct to Play Will Make Our Children Happier, More Self-Reliant, and Better Students for Life.* Basic Books 2015

Greene, Robert: *Mastery.* Profile Books 2012

Helmstetter, Shad: *What to Say When You Talk to Yourself.* Thorsons 1991

Holiday, Ryan: *The Obstacle is the Way: The Ancient Art of Turning Adversity to Advantage.* Profile Books 2015

Joseph, Stephen: *Authentic: How to Be Yourself and Why It Matters.* Piatkus 2019

Koch, Richard: *The 80/20 Principle: Achieve More with Less.* Nicholas Brealey Publishing 2022

Bibliography

Linden, David J.: *Unique: The New Science of Human Individuality.* Basic Books 2020

Loehr, Jim: *The Power of Full Engagement: Managing Energy, Not Time, Is the Key to High Performance and Personal Renewal.* Simon & Schuster 2005

McGonigal, Kelly: *The Willpower Instinct: How Self-Control Works, Why It Matters, and What You Can Do to Get More of It.* Avery Publishing Group 2013

McGraw, Phillip C.: *Life Strategies: The No-Nonsense Approach to Turning Your Life Around.* Vermilion 2001

Rankin, Lissa: *The Fear Cure: Cultivating Courage as Medicine for the Body, Mind, and Soul.* Hay House 2015

Ryan, M.J.: *How to Survive Change . . . You Didn't Ask For: Bounce Back, Find Calm in Chaos, and Reinvent Yourself.* Conari Press 2014

Ryan, M.J.: *The Power of Patience: How This Old-Fashioned Virtue Can Improve Your Life.* Conrari Press 2021

Thaler, Richard and Sunstein, Cass: *Nudge: Improving Decisions About Health, Wealth and Happiness.* Allen Lane 2021

Habits

Carr, Allen: *Allen Carr's Easy Way to Stop Smoking.* Penguin Books 2015

Clear, James: *Atomic Habits: An Easy & Proven Way to Build Good Habits & Break Bad Ones.* Random House Business 2018

Covey, Stephen R.: *The 7 Habits of Highly Effective People.* Simon & Schuster 2020

Duhigg, Charles: *The Power of Habit: Why We Do What We Do, and How to Change.* Random House Books 2013

Sleep

Foster, Russell: *Life Time: The New Science of the Body Clock, and How It Can Revolutionize Your Sleep and Health.* Penguin Life 2022

Panda, Satchin: *The Circadian Code: Lose Weight, Supercharge Your Energy and Sleep Well Every Night.* Vermilion 2018

Strand, Clark: *Waking Up to the Dark: The Black Madonna's Gospel for an Age of Extinction and Collapse.* Monkfish Book Publishing 2022

Walker, Matthew: *Why We Sleep: The New Science of Sleep and Dreams.* Penguin 2018

Diet and nutrition

Bikman, Benjamin: *Why We Get Sick: The Hidden Epidemic at the Root of Most Chronic Disease – and How to Fight It.* Benbella Books 2021

Blaser, Martin: *Missing Microbes: How Killing Bacteria Creates Modern Plagues.* Oneworld Publications 2015

Eenfeldt, Andreas: *Low Carb, High Fat Food Revolution: Advice and Recipes to Improve Your Health and Reduce Your Weight.* Skyhorse Publishing 2017

Fung, Jason with Moore, Jimmy: *The Complete Guide to Fasting: Heal Your Body Through Intermittent, Alternate-Day, and Extended Fasting.* Victory Belt Publishing 2016

Lustig, Robert: *Metabolical: The Truth About Processed Food and How it Poisons People and the Planet.* Yellow Kite 2021

Pelz, Mindy: *Fast Like a Girl: A Woman's Guide to Using the Healing Power of Fasting to Burn Fat, Boost Energy, and Balance Hormones.* Hay House 2022

Pollan, Michael: *Food Rules: An Eater's Manual.* Penguin 2010

Spector, Tim: *Spoon-Fed: Why Almost Everything We've Been Told About Food is Wrong.* Vintage 2022

Yong, Ed: *I Contain Multitudes: The Microbes Within Us and a Grander View of Life.* Vintage 2017

Van Tulleken, Chris: *Ultra-Processed People: Why Do We All Eat Stuff That Isn't Food . . . and Why Can't We Stop?* Cornerstone Press 2023

Movement and exercise

Arnot, Bob: *Flip the Youth Switch.* iBooks 2020

Hansen, Anders: *The Real Happy Pill: Power Up Your Brain by Moving Your Body.* Skyhorse Publishing 2017

Bibliography

Lieberman, Daniel: *Exercised: The Science of Physical Activity, Rest and Health*. Allen Lane 2020

McGonigal, Kelly: *The Joy of Movement: How Exercise Helps Us Find Happiness, Hope, Connection, and Courage*. Avery Publishing Group 2020

Ratey, John R. and Hagerman, Eric: *Spark: How Exercise Will Improve the Performance of Your Brain*. Quercus 2010

Stress

Chatterjee, Rangan: *The Stress Solution: The 4 Steps to a Calmer, Happier, Healthier You*. Penguin Life 2018

Epel, Elissa: *The Seven-Day Stress Prescription*. Penguin Life 2022

Maté, Gabor: *When the Body Says No: The Cost of Hidden Stress*. Vermilion 2019

McGonigal, Kelly: *The Upside of Stress: Why Stress Is Good for You (and How to Get Good At It)*. Vermilion 2015

Selye, Hans: *Stress Without Distress*. Jenson Books 1975

Selye, Hans: *The Stress of Life*. McGraw-Hill 1978

Active rest

Hammond, Claudia: *The Art of Rest: How to Find Respite in the Modern Age*. Canongate Books 2020

Harper, Mark: *Chill – The Cold Water Swim Cure*. Chronicle Books 2022

Hof, Wim: *The Wim Hof Method: Activate Your Potential, Transcend Your Limits*. Rider 2022

Holiday, Ryan: *Stillness Is the Key: An Ancient Strategy for Modern Life*. Profile Books 2019

Kagge, Erling: *Silence: In the Age of Noise*. Penguin Books 2018

Lagos, Leah: *Heart Breath Mind: Conquer Stress, Build Resilience, and Perform at Your Peak*. Harvest Publications 2021

Nestor, James: *Breath: The New Science of a Lost Art*. Penguin Life 2021

Nichols, Wallace J.: *Blue Mind: How Water Makes You Happier, More Connected and Better at What You Do*. Abacus 2018

Tolle, Eckhart: *The Power of Now: A Guide to Spiritual Enlightenment*. Yellow Kite 2001

Williams, Florence: *The Nature Fix: Why Nature Makes Us Happier, Healthier, and More Creative*. W.W. Norton & Company 2018

Alcohol
Turner, Sara and Rocca, Lucy: *The Sober Revolution: Women Calling Time on Wine O'Clock*. Accent Press 2015

Lifestyle
Buettner, Dan: *The Blue Zones: Lessons for Living Longer from the People Who've Lived Longest*. National Geographic Society 2010
Chatterjee, Rangan: *The 4 Pillar Plan: How to Relax, Eat, Move and Sleep Your Way to a Longer, Healthier Life*. Penguin Life 2017
Rankin, Lissa: *Mind Over Medicine: Scientific Proof That You Can Heal Yourself*. Hay House 2020